RECENT ADVANCES IN THE FIELD OF URINARY TRACT INFECTIONS

Edited by **Thomas Nelius**

Recent Advances in the Field of Urinary Tract Infections
http://dx.doi.org/10.5772/46044
Edited by Thomas Nelius

Contributors

Mohamed Labib, Nenad Spasojevic, Yusuf Kibar, Maja Zivkovic, Ljiljana Stojkovic, Brankica Spasojevic-Dimitrijeva, Mirjana Milorad Kostic, Aleksandra Stankovic, Kumar Venkitanarayanan, Mary Anne Roshni Amalaradjou, Vivian Yeefong Leung, Winnie Chiu Wing Chu, Thomas Nelius, Christopher Winter, Stephanie Filleur, Leslie Kammire, Skrepetis Kostadinos, Efthimiou Ioannis

Published by InTech
Janeza Trdine 9, 51000 Rijeka, Croatia

Publishing Process Manager Sandra Bakic
Technical Editor InTech DTP team
Cover InTech Design team

Additional hard copies can be obtained from orders@intechopen.com

Recent Advances in the Field of Urinary Tract Infections, Edited by Thomas Nelius
p. cm.
ISBN 978-953-51-1180-1

For EU product safety concerns:
IN TECH d.o.o., Prolaz Marije Krucifikse Kozulić 3, 51000 Rijeka, Croatia,
info@intechopen.com or visit our website at intechopen.com.

Meet the editor

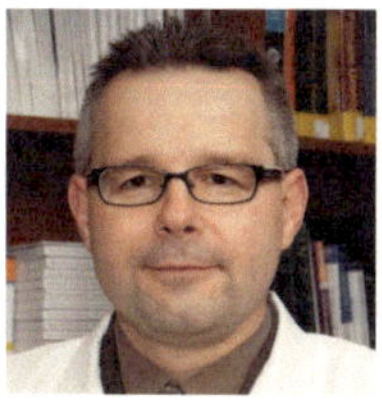

Thomas Nelius was born in Aschersleben, Germany, in 1967. He received the Medical Degree and Doctor of Philosophy from the University Halle/Wittenberg, Germany in 1994 and 1995, respectively. He completed his Residency in Urology at a Teaching Hospital of the Otto-von-Guericke University Magdeburg, Germany and at the Princess of Wales Hospital, Bridgend, United Kingdom from 1994-2000. He is Board Certified by the German Board of Urology. From 2001-2003, he was a Research Associate of the Department of Urology at Northwestern University Chicago, IL, USA, where he worked on the development of new anti-angiogenic treatment strategies. Presently, he is an Associate Professor in the Department of Urology at Texas Tech University Health Sciences Center, Lubbock, TX, USA. His area of expertise includes also treatment of urological malignancies. He is mainly interested in new treatment strategies for prostate cancer, including e.g. anti-angiogenic strategies and metronomic chemotherapy in patients with hormone-refractory prostate cancer. He is an active reviewer for multiple Medical Journals and and member of the American Urological Association, German Society of Urology, South Central Section of the American Urological Association, American Society of Clinical Oncology, American Association of Cancer Research and Southwest Oncology Group Affiliate Program.

Contents

Preface

Urinary tract infections (UTI) continue to be under the most common bacterial infections worldwide. Diagnostic and treatment have substantial financial burden on society. In the USA, UTIs are responsible for more than 7 million physician visits annually and about 15% of all community-prescribed antibiotics in the USA are dispensed for UTIs. About 50% of women will experience at least one UTI episode during lifetime, about 1 million emergency department visits due to UTI in the USA alone, resulting in more than 100 000 hospital admissions annually, most often for pyelonephritis. Moreover, UTIs are also the leading cause of hospital-acquired infections, accounting for approximately 40% of all such cases. The majority of these cases are catheter-associated. Therefore, nosocomial UTIs comprise perhaps the largest institutional reservoir for nosocomial antibiotic-resistant pathogens. Beside the economic impact, UTIs affect also significantly the quality of life of the affected population. The aim of this book is to highlight problematic aspects and recent advances in the field of UTIs. The book is divided in three parts.

The first part covers issues regarding catheter-associated UTIs including prevention, problems in developing countries and the role of bacterial biofilms.

In the second part deals with potential new diagnostic developments for pediatric related UTIs. This includes new concepts regarding dysfunctional voiding and new anatomical aspects of the vesico-ureteral junction.

Genetic factors underlying susceptibility upper UTIs and potential immune-based treatment strategies are discussed in the third part of the book.

Thomas Nelius
Texas Tech University Health Sciences Center,
Department of Urology,
Lubbock, Texas
United States of America

Section 1

Management of Catheter-Associated Urinary Tract Infections

Chapter 1

Prevention of Urinary Tract Infections in the Outpatient and Inpatient Settings

Leslie Kammire

Additional information is available at the end of the chapter

http://dx.doi.org/10.5772/56709

1. Introduction

Urinary tract infections (UTIs) are one of the most common health problems plaguing women. About half of women will experience a UTI during their lifetime. The incidence is much lower in men but increases with age. In patients over the age of 65, at least 20% of women and 10% of men have bacteruria [1]. The incidence also increases with hospitalization or institutionalization. UTIs are the most common nosocomial infection, and more than 80% of these are associated with an indwelling catheter [2]. There is also a higher risk of UTIS in pregnancy and some chronic diseases including diabetes, multiple sclerosis, spinal cord injuries or disease, and immunosuppressive diseases such as HIV.

The cost of treating UTIs is substantial both in inpatient and outpatient settings. In the United States in the year 2007, approximately 2.47 billion dollars were spent on outpatient treatment of UTI and this excluded spending on prescriptions [3]. The estimated cost of nosocomial UTIS is approximately 2.66 billion dollars in 2007 dollars [4]. There are simple and effective measures for prevention of UTIs which can significantly limit morbidity and cost, but these are often overlooked,

Certain patients, particularly women, despite having normal anatomy and function of the urinary tract, are genetically predisposed to urinary tract infections. This tendency seems to be related to variations in the urinary tract epithelium and it's interaction with bacteria. Once a person has a UTI, he or she is more likely to get another within a year. Recurrence rates in women vary from 28 to 82%, with higher rates seen in women with a prior history of UTI [5]. The risk of recurrent UTIs increases with higher number of prior infections. It also decreases with a longer time interval between the first and second infections. [4] However, even with long intervals between infections, about one sixth of women have difficulties with recurrent infections throughout their lifetime [4]. Preventive strategies should be targeted to this group.

2. Prevention of UTIS in the outpatient setting

Given the increasing emergence of multidrug resistant bacteria in UTIs, every effort should be made to use non-pharmacologic measures as first line preventive strategies in patient who have recurrent UTIs.

2.1. Hygiene

There are many "old wives" tales about causes of UTIs, and many of these beliefs are ingrained in women. Women are told by other women to wear cotton underwear, avoid drinking sodas, and even to avoid strong laundry detergent in an effort to prevent UTIS.

Studies have not been done to evaluate most of these measures. A search of PubMed using the terms "urinary tract infection" and "sodas, carbonated beverages, hygiene, wiping patterns" did not reveal any studies. However, it is intuitive that girls and women should always wipe from front to back after a bowel movement to avoid brining fecal bacteria towards the vagina and the urethra. If a woman is predisposed to urinary tract infections, she should carefully watch hygiene. It is helpful to show these women a picture of the vulvar anatomy, explaining the close proximity of the urethra to the anal area and that an infection occurs when intestinal bacteria enter the urethra. These women should be encouraged to clean with a moist wipe (such as a baby wipe or other hygienic cleansing wipe) after a bowel movement. It is the author's opinion that it is helpful to wash the perineum and perianal area with antibacterial soap prior to intercourse. Patients should also be instructed to avoid any sexual practices that might bring colonic bacteria forward towards the vagina, such as touching the perianal area and then the vaginal area. Voiding after intercourse has been shown to protect against UTI [5]. There is no evidence that vaginal douching after intercourse decreases UTI incidence and in fact, it may increase the risk of vaginal infections. As such, it is not a recommended practice.

It is also the author's opinion that patient with recurrent UTIs should avoid tub baths. This recommendation comes from repeated observations over years of practice that many women who present UTIs give a history of taking frequent tub baths. It is plausible that the hot water washes away some of the protective mucous coating the urethral and vaginal introitus, making the mucosa drier and more susceptible to bacterial colonization. There were no studies on this found during a literature search on PupMed and OVID using the search terms "tub bath" "bathing" and "urinary tract infection". There were interestingly a few papers in the 70s linking Pseudomonas infections, including UTIs, to whirlpools and hot tubs, and this led the Centers for Disease Control (CDC) in the United States to establish standards for chlorination and filtration of these tubs [6]. Patient with UTIs should likely avoid these public tubs as well. Even if the water is correctly chlorinated and filtered, it is extremely hot and drying to the skin.

2.2. Diet

There is evidence that links overactive bladder but not UTI to regular consumption of carbonated beverages. A large study that examined the prevalence and incidence of irritative voiding symptoms in men and women over a 12 months period showed a significant association between onset of overactive bladder and weekly consumption of carbonated drinks. (P=. 03). These findings did not apply to men in the survey [7]. There are also several studies linking caffeine to lower urinary tract symptoms, but not infection [8], [9].

Although these data don't indicate that dietary factors actually cause UTIS, women who have frequent UTIs often mistake the frequency and urgency caused by a dietary bladder irritant for an infection. This could lead to calls to their provider requesting therapy and the chance of overtreatment. Thus it would seem prudent for these women who are plagued with frequent UTIS to avoid an excessive amount of carbonated beverages and caffeine. There may well be other dietary bladder irritants, such as citrus and other acidic fruits that can cause urgency. It is helpful for women with frequent UTIS to keep a food diary for a short time and see if they can link certain foods to irritative voiding symptoms.

2.3. Contraception

Although there are no contraceptive methods that prevent UTIs, there are several that may increase the risk, primarily diaphragms and spermicides. Diaphragms were widely used in the 1950s through the early 1980s, but are not often used now that there are more effective methods of contraception that are easier to use. Diaphragm users have been shown to have a two to threefold increased risk of UTI compared to non-users [10], [11]. This is due to partial urethral compression by the rim of the diaphragm and also is likely related to the spermicide that is used on the rim.

Spermicides contain nonoxynol-9 which can cause a chemical irritation to the vaginal and urethral mucosa as well as changes in the normal flora. This in turn predisposes to colonization by coliforms as well as Staph saprophyticus [12]. Patients with recurrent UTIs should avoid diaphragms and spermicide coated condoms, as well as other barrier agents containing nonoxynol-9 such as foam, suppositories, and sponges.

2.4. Vaginal estrogen replacement for postmenopausal women

After menopause, the vulvar skin atrophies and thins. There is decreased blood flow to this area and decreased mucous production. The periurethral mucosa is lubricated by the Skene's glands and these also atrophy, thus causing loss of mucous that is the first line of defense against bacteria. In addition, vaginal ph increases after menopause and lactobacilli counts decrease. These conditions set up the postmenopausal woman for higher risk of UTIs, particularly after intercourse. In addition, urinary incontinence, the presence of a cystocele and incomplete emptying and have been found to be highly associated with recurrent UTI, and these are problems that increase with age as well [13].

Systemic estrogen replacement therapy in the prevention of UTI has not been shown to be of help in preventing recurrent UTIs in postmenopausal women. However, there is strong evidence that *topical vaginal* estrogen replacement does protect against recurrent UTIs. Raz and Stamm in 1993 conducted a randomized controlled trial in postmenopausal women and found a significant decrease in rate of urinary tract infections in the treated group which used intravaginal estrogen twice weekly, versus placebo., (0.5 vs. 5.9 episodes per patient-year,

P<0.001. They demonstrated a return of lactobacilli to the vaginal flora and normalization of vaginal ph. In addition, vaginal colonization with Enterobacteriaceae fell from 67 percent to 31% in the treated group [13].

Vaginal estrogen therapy is available in three forms in the United States. These are listed in decreasing order of systemic absorption:

1. Estradiol vaginal cream: Premarin Vaginal cream = 0.625 mg/gm and Estrace vaginal cream = 0.1 mg/gm. Dosage varies from 0.5 mg to 2 mg/vagina twice weekly. Retail cost is $140/tube for both of these products (www.drugstore.com)

2. Estradiol vaginal tablets: Vagifem = 10 mcg estrogen per tablet. Dosage is one tablet inserted vaginally twice weekly. Retail cost is $64.00/month

3. Estradiol 2 mg vaginal ring. One ring is placed intravaginally and changed every 3 months. Retail cost is $216.00 per ring (3 months).

An exact dosage for vaginal estrogen therapy for UTI prevention hasn't been established. Raz's landmark study used 0.5 mg estriol cream intravaginally once daily for 2 weeks, then twice weekly. Estriol cream is not commercially available in the United States and most prescribers use one to two grams of Estrace or Premarin cream per vagina twice weekly. Dosage should be individualized based on patient weight and degree of atrophy present. In an obese woman with higher levels of endogenous estrogen, 0.5 mg of estrogen cream twice weekly will likely be adequate, whereas in a thin woman who is very atrophic, a higher dose will be needed, especially in the initial months of treatment. Of note, progesterone does not need to be prescribed with topical vaginal estrogen in women with a uterus. In the recommended dosages, vaginal estrogen therapy does not cause endometrial hyperplasia as the amount of systemic absorption of estrogen is quite low. Progesterone therapy does NOT need to be given in a woman with a uterus who is using vaginal estrogen on a long term basis.

Despite strong evidence of benefit, topical estrogen is underutilized as a preventive strategy. In a study of nursing home residents in Norway who were on preventive therapy for UTI, only about 10% were prescribed vaginal estrogen [14]. Many women have a fear of estrogen containing products due to fear of breast or uterine cancer. There is no evidence that vaginal estrogen therapy causes uterine cancer or even endometrial hyperplasia. The same holds true for breast cancer. Patients often need reassurance that vaginal estrogen is safe and doesn't have the risk of systemic ERT, which uses much higher dosages. Vaginal estrogen therapy can be used safely in women with a prior history of breast cancer or thrombosis. The estrogen ring has the lowest amount of systemic absorption, followed by the vaginal estrogen tablets, then cream.

Cost is also significant obstacle in the United States, as many health insurance plans don't cover these products well, and after age 65 there is variable coverage of these with Medicare. One solution for women who cannot afford these products is to have a compounding pharmacist make an equivalent substitute. Estradiol 0.1 mg/gm can be added to a pluronic gel base that has excellent adherence to the vaginal mucosa. Cost is approximately $50.00 for a two to three month supply.

2.5. Natural remedies

Cranberries and their juice have long been touted for both treatment and prevention of UTI. This was previously thought to be due to acidification of the urine, but more recent research has shown that substances (proanthocyanadins) in the cranberry prevent adhesion of E. coli strains to the uroepithelium, including multidrug resistant strains [15]. Studies of cranberry prophylaxis are mixed, but several recent studies have shown that there is benefit from this simple remedy. Wang et al did a meta-analysis of randomized controlled trials comparing prevention of UTIs in users of cranberry products versus placebo or non-placebo controls. They found a risk ratio for cranberry users versus nonusers was 0.62 and statistically significant, leading them to conclude that cranberry products are associated with protection against UTIs. Further, cranberry products were more effective in certain subgroups including women with recurrent UTIs, children, cranberry juice users (as opposed to tablets) and those who used cranberry products more than twice daily [16].

A recent RCT examined women with recurrent UTIs, randomizing them to either cranberry juice or placebo for 6 months. Those in the cranberry juice did have lower incidence of recurrent UTIS, but it did not reach statistical significance. However, they did have significantly decreased counts of P-fimbriated E. coli in their urine during the study periods. These are uropathogenic strains with fimbriae capable of attaching to the uroepethelium. The authors concluded that though the cranberry juice didn't significant reduce the number of recurrent UTIs, the reduction in adherent E. coli lends plausibility to a protective effect of cranberry and warrants further large scale studies [17].

Within the pediatric population, several new cranberry studies have emerged. A RCT from Finland randomized 263 children with a prior history of UTI to 6 months of cranberry juice versus placebo. Their findings: the juice did not significantly reduce the number of children who experienced a recurrence of UTI, but it was effective in reducing the actual number of recurrences and related antimicrobial use [18]. Another recent randomized controlled prospective study found cranberry capsules effective in the prevention of UTI in children with neurogenic bladder caused by myelomeningocele who required chronic intermittent catheterization. The median UTI rate in this small cohort of 20 children was 0.5 UTI/year during placebo usage and 0/year with cranberry capsule usage. This decrease was statistically significant. No side effects were noted [19].

Cranberry juice is safe in pregnancy and there is data from a small study to suggest that it may be efficacious in preventing asyptomatic bacteruria and symptomatic UTI. However in this same study, the juice was poorly tolerated by the pregnant women, and there was a high rate of withdrawal [20]. If used in pregnancy, use of cranberry pill form will likely be more effective as compliance will be higher.

Propolis is a resinous material collected by bees from exudates and buds of plants, then mixed with wax and bee enzymes. It has well documented antibacterial activity. Lavigne et al added propolis to proanthocyanidins from the cranberry and studied its effect on human volunteer subjects. They found that once daily ingestion offers some protection against bacterial adhesion, bacterial multiplication and virulence in the urinary tract [21].

Blueberries and blackberries are widely touted on the internet as effective prevention for UTIs but there are no trials of these foods found on PubMed or Ovid. Bearberry leaves are another folk remedy believed to be helpful in treating mild UTIs, but likewise, no studies of effectiveness have been undertaken. The same hold true for Vitamin C. There are no studies of this alone for prevention of UTI. However when Vitamin C was added to cranberry extract, D-mannose, fructo-oligosaccharides, and bromelain, this mixture was effective in reducing recurrent UTIs and improving quality of life in both pre and postmenopausal women [22]. More studies are needed on efficacy of these nutraceuticals.

In summary, there is emerging evidence that cranberries are effective in the prevention of UTI in women and children, including children with neurogenic bladder. Both the juice and the capsules seem to be effective, the juice possibly more so, but it should be unsweetened juice to prevent high intake of unnecessary sugars. The capsules may be better tolerated however, particularly in pregnancy. Whichever form is used, it seems that it should be ingested three or more times daily for maximal effectiveness. The optimal dose of cranberry is not known and was studied in only one of the studies included in Wang's meta-analysis [23]. He concluded that the cranberry juice provides the most benefit, and it should be ingested three times daily at a dose of 4 to 6 ounces [24]. Most over the counter cranberry preperations contain 400 to 500 mg of cranberry extract and are likely also more effective if taken three times/daily. More studies are needed in this area to determine the optimal dose and type of cranberry. Cranberries should be used with caution in patients on blood thinners and those with kidney stones.

2.6. Vaccines

Attempts have been underway to create an oral or parental immunoprophylaxis or vaccination for patients with recurrent UTIs for some time, but these efforts have been frustrated by the short lived nature of immunity created. The premise of a vaccine is inactivated bacteria or bacterial components presented to a host's mucosal surface to boost immunity. Intransal sprays, sublingual preparations, vaginal suppositories and IM injections have been developed thus far. Recent publications show promise in this area. Currently, a vaccine has been developed by Immunotek in Spain called Uromune® a sublingual preparation which contains an inactivated bacterial cell suspension of selected strains of *Escherichia coli, Klebsiella pneumoniae, Proteus vulgaris,* and *Enterococcus faecalis*. A multicenter observational study was conducted by Lorenzo-Gomez et al in which a group of 319 women with a history of recurrent UTIs were divided into two groups. Group A was treated with 3 months of this vaccine and Group B with 6 months of prophylactic antibiotic treatment with sulfamethoxazole/trimethoprim 200/40 mg/day. These women were then followed for 15 months. The authors found that patients in Group A had a highly statistically significant decrease in number of UTI's that persisted for up to 15 months. The numbers of patients who did not have any UTI at 3, 9, and 15 months were 101, 90, and 55 in group A versus 9, 4, and 0 in group B ($P < 0.0001$) [25].

2.7. Pharmacologic suppressive treatments: Antibacterial

2.7.1. Methenamine hippurate

Methenamine hippurate is not an antibiotic, but is a urinary antibacterial agent used for prevention of recurrent UTI when long term therapy is needed. It exhibits antibacterial activity by conversion of methenamine to formaldehyde in the presence of acidic urine. The hippuric acid component acidifies the urine and also has some antibacterial activity. This drug is often used in combination with a urinary acidifier such as sodium phosphate (Uroqid acid#2). The dose for suppression is 1 gram orally twice daily. It is safe for both adult and pediatric patients, but is contraindicated in patients with renal or hepatic insufficiency. Methenamine is Pregnancy Category C, and there are no adequate and well controlled studies of its use in pregnancy. It is excreted in breast milk and the amount excreted does not appear to adversely affect the nursing infant.

Methenamine is effective in the prevention of recurrent UTIs in both adult and pediatric patients, but should only be used following eradication of the infection by antibiotics. It is not as effective as nitrofurantoin or trimethoprim/sulfamethoxazole as prophylactic treatment, but also does not cause antimicrobial resistance. Per Micromedex, it has shown to be effective in reducing bacteruria in gynecological surgical patients with short term foley catheter placement up to 3 days, but was not effective in prophylaxis for patients with long term indwelling catheters.

Most of the studies of efficacy of methenamine were done in the 1960s and 70's. Lee et al undertook a meta-analysis of all studies in 2007. There were 13 studies included, 6 of which reported on symptomatic UTI and eight for bacteruria. The overall estimates were difficult to interpret due to heterogeneity of the studies. Subgroup analysis did show that methenamine likely has benefit in patients without renal tract abnormalities for both symptomatic UTI and bacteruria but not in patients with known renal tract abnormalities. The authors concluded that methenamine may be effective for preventing UTI in patients without rental tract abnormalities, especially when used for short-term prophylaxis. It doesn't appear to work in patients with neurogenic bladder or those who have renal tract abnormalities. The rate of adverse events is low. There is a need for further large well RCT to clarify the value of its longer term use for patients without renal tract abnormalities [26].

2.8. Pharmacologic suppressive treatments: Antimicrobials

There are 3 strategies commonly used today for prevention for patients with recurrent UTI:

1. Post coital therapy: The patient takes a single dose of an antibiotic immediately after intercourse

2. Patient initiated therapy: The patient takes a single antibiotic tablet on first noticing symptoms of infection

3. Continuous daily suppression: The patient takes a daily dose of suppressive antibiotic for 3 to 6 months or sometimes longer.

Choosing an effective preventive strategy should be individualized and keep in mind the ultimate goal to minimize exposure to long term antibiotics. Regardless, it should be noted that a patient will improve during any of these types of suppressive therapy, but once therapy is discontinued, the patient's risk of recurrent UTIs increases back to baseline. This again underscores the need for more effective long-term preventive strategies.

For those women who find sexual intercourse to commonly trigger an infection, post-coital therapy would be the easiest and safest option. Patient initiated therapy has been used for many years and is most beneficial for women who have infrequent or clustered recurrent UTIs. Adherent and motivated patients have been shown to be able to accurately self diagnose UTIs 95% of the time and successfully self treat with a short course of antibiotics taken at onset of symptoms [27]. Zhong et al found that patient-initiated single-dose intermittent antibiotic prophylaxis was as effective as low-dose daily antibiotic prophylaxis in the treatment of recurrent UTIs in post menopausal women and was associated with fewer gastrointestinal side effects [28].

Finally, continuous daily suppression has been shown in numerous studies to effectively reduce the incidence of recurrent UTIs by up to 95%. However, in an effort to decrease development of resistance, the first two options are recommended as initial therapy. This option should be reserved for those patients who don't respond to intermittent therapy or are unable to be compliant with it. Most clinicians treat for a 6 month period, but in patients who continue to have frequent episodes, longer periods varying from 2 to 5 years have been used.

The antibiotics most commonly used in suppressive therapies are nitrofurantoin, trimethoprim (TMP), trimethoprim with sulfamethoxazole (TMP/SMX), and fosfomycin. Quinolones or first generation cephalosporins were also used in some trials, but given their broader spectrum of action, they should NOT be used as prophylactic therapy. None of these antibiotics has shown superior effectiveness in UTI prophylaxis.

Nitrofurantoin is an attractive first choice as its bactericidal action is limited to the urinary tract. The dose most often used for prophylaxis is 50 to 100 mg/day, taken after intercourse or at bedtime with food. Once ingested, it has a very short half life in serum (about 30 minutes) and is excreted into the urine. It is effective against *Escherichia coli, Enterococcus, Staphylococcus aureus,* as well as some strains of *Klebsiella* and *Enterobacter*. Due to multiple sites of action, resistance has not been a problem despite over 55 years of use. Nitrofurantoin is not associated with impaired fertility or teratogenicity and is considered safe in pregnancy and breastfeeding. It has few drug interactions, making it an attractive choice for treating elderly patients on multiple medications. It should not be used in patients with impaired renal function. Primary side effects are nausea, emesis and anorexia [29].

Despite its overall safety, rare but serious adverse effects are reported. The most widely known is pulmonary toxicity [29]. Reports also exist of toxic hepatitis and blood dyscrasias [29]. Neurotoxicity from nitrofurantoin is less recognized, and is estimated to occur in 0.0007 percent of courses of therapy [29]. *All of these toxicities can be severe or even fatal, and their occurrence is independent of the length of time the drug is taken. Because these side effects are rare, practitioners who prescribe suppressive therapy with nitrofurantoin must be aware of these.*

http://dx.doi.org/10.5772/56709

Fosfomycin tromethamine is a powder mixed with four ounces of water and drank. It is supplied in a sachet containing 3 grams. The dose is 3 gram as a one-time treatment of uncomplicated UTI. It has also been shown to be highly effective in prophylaxis of UTI recurrence at a dose of 3 grams every 10 days [30]. There is no data on its use as post-coital therapy. It inhibits bacterial cell wall synthesis and also decreases bacterial adherence of to the urothelium. It is most active against Staphylococci (including *S. Saprophiticus*) and *E. coli*, as well as some strains of *Pseudomonas* and *Proteus*. It is less active against enterococci, *Klebsiella spp, Enterobacter* and *Proteus mirabilis*. Good in vitro activity is reported against methicillin-resistant *S. aureus* (MRSA). It is Pregnancy Category B and is safe in pregnancy and breast-feeding. Side effects are mostly minor, including rash, nausea and diarrhea, headache, and back pain. There are rare reports in Drugdex of hepatic toxicity.

TMP-SMX has long been used as suppressive therapy and is effective. There is not much data on the effectiveness of Trimethoprim alone. The dose is trimethoprim 40 mg/sulfamethoxazole 200 mg either after intercourse, three times weekly, or daily. It is Pregnancy Category C but is considered safe to use in pregnancy, though if alternatives are available, another agent is recommended in the first trimester due to the folic acid anatagonist activity of trimethoprim. It is also considered safe to use during breastfeeding. Increasing resistance to this agent should be noted. In the recent Antimicrobial Resistance Epidemiology in Females with Cystitis (ARSEC) study in nine European countries and Brazil, 30-50% of all isolated urinary pathogens were resistant to TMP-SMX [31]. Side effects of TMP-SMX are common and primary gastro-intestinal: nausea, emesis and anorexia. Rash is also common. Rarely, more serious side effects occur such as Stevens-Johnson syndrome, toxic epidermal necrolysis or aplastic anemia.

3. Prevention of UTIS in the inpatient and institutional setting

UTIS are the most common nosocomial infection worldwide, accounting for about 40% of these. The great majority of these infections are due to the presence of an indwelling urethral catheter in hospitals and long-term care facilities (LTCF) and are commonly referred to as catheter-associated UTI (CAUTI). These infections add significantly to morbidity and sometimes even mortality for the patient. The cost of these infections is substantial, estimated at 2.66 billion dollars in 2007 US dollars [32].

More than 1.5 million people in the United States live in nursing homes. Within the last decade, the severity of illness of nursing home residents has increased such that these residents (average age 80) have a risk of developing health care-associated infection (HAI) that approaches that seen hospital inpatients. The use of indwelling foley catheters has decreased in this setting and is currently about 5 to 10%, but UTI remains the leading infection in long term care facilities (LTCFs). Guidelines for prevention of CA-UTI applies to both these settings [33]. Of note, the catheter literature commonly reports on catheter-associated asymptomatic bacteruria (CA-ASB) and catheter associated bacteruria if no distinction is made between CA-ASB and CA-UTI. CA-bacteruria is the predominant outcome measure reported in most clinical trials.

Undoubtedly, the best way to prevent UTI is to avoid long term catheterization. The risk of UTI goes up markedly about 72 hours after a foley catheter is inserted. As long term foley use is often unavoidable in the hospitalized or nursing home patient, much attention has been devoted to efforts to prevent CAUTI worldwide. The Department of Public Health in England developed guidelines in 2001 and updated them in 2007 [34]. A short time later, in 2008 the European Association of Urology (EAU), the Urological Association of Asia (UAA), and others published *European and Asian Guidelines on Management and Prevention of Catheter-Associated Urinary Tract [35].* Within the United States, the Center for Disease Control (CDC) first published guidelines in 1981 and these have been intermittently revised, most recently in 2009 [36]. During this same year, the the Infectious Diseases Society of America published guidelines for the diagnosis, prevention and treatment of CAUTI as well [37].

Recently Conway and Larsen reviewed and compared a total of 8 guidelines worldwide to prevent CAUTI. They found broad agreement between the guidelines overall but noted that different grading systems for the level of evidence to support each recommendation made comparisons difficult. They also noted that most of the guidelines didn't distinguish between true catheter associated infections as opposed to catheter associated asymptomatic bacteruria. They wisely noted that "For clinicians seeking to prevent CAUTI, the distinction is a moot point, because all symptomatic CAUTI begins as asymptomatic bacteruria". Their article included an excellent, concise summary of all 8 of these guidelines. This included an overview of recommendations for catheter use, catheter types, insertion techniques, maintenance, and antimicrobials [38].

Within the United States, the guidelines for prevention are very similar between the CDC and ISDA 2009 guidelines. These guidelines are summarized below. The ISDA guidelines note that most of their recommendations pertain to the prevention of catheter-associated bacteruria as this is the reported outcome in most trials, whereas the CDC doesn't differentiate between bacteruria and symptomatic UTI. Both guidelines provided evidence for strength of each recommendation. The CDC evidence levels were used in this summary and are defined in Table 1. They are noted in blue.

Category IA	A strong recommendation supported by high to moderate quality† evidence suggesting net clinical benefits or harms
Category IB	A strong recommendation supported by low quality evidence suggesting net clinical benefits or harms or an accepted practice (e.g., aseptic technique) supported by low to very low quality evidence
Category IC	A strong recommendation required by state or federal regulation.
Category II	A weak recommendation supported by any quality evidence suggesting a trade off between clinical benefits and harms
No recommendation/ unresolved issue	Unresolved issue for which there is low to very low quality evidence with uncertain trade offs between benefits and harms

Table 1. Modified HICPAC Categorization Scheme* for Recommendations (Reprinted from CDC [39]).

4. Recommendations for the prevention of CAUTI indications for use

- Insert catheter only for appropriate indications (see Table 2) and leave in place only as long as needed (Category 1B)

Catheters should NOT be placed for incontinence or nursing convenience. For the postoperative patient who needs an indwelling catheter, remove within 24 hours unless there are indications for continued use, such as surgery on the urinary tract or an open perineal wound. Then remember to remove as soon as medically feasible. The use of condom catheters in incontinent male patients should be considered but this is considered an unresolved issue due to insufficient data.

Patient has acute urinary retention or bladder outlet obstruction
Need for accurate measurements of urinary output in critically ill patients
Perioperative use for selected surgical procedures: 1. Patients undergoing urologic surgery or other surgery on contiguous structures of the genitourinary tract 2. Anticipated prolonged duration of surgery (catheters inserted for this reason should be removed in PACU) 3. Patients anticipated to receive large-volume infusions or diuretics during surgery 4. Need for intraoperative monitoring of urinary output
To assist in healing of open sacral or perineal wounds in incontinent patients
Patient requires prolonged immobilization (e.g., potentially unstable thoracic or lumbar spine, multiple traumatic injuries such as pelvic fractures)
To improve comfort for end of life care if needed
B. Examples of Inappropriate Uses of Indwelling Catheters
As a substitute for nursing care of the patient or resident with incontinence
As a means of obtaining urine for culture or other diagnostic tests when the patient can voluntarily void
For prolonged postoperative duration without appropriate indications (e.g., structural repair of urethra or contiguous structures, prolonged effect of epidural anaesthesia, etc.)

Table 2. Examples of Appropriate Indications for Indwelling Urethral Catheter Use (Reprinted from CDC [39]).

- Use alternative to indwelling catheters when appropriate

  – Condom catheters in male patients without obstruction or retention (Category II). The use of condom catheters vs indwelling catheter has been studied in a randomized controlled trial of hospitalized men aged 40 and over. Results showed condom catheter use is less likely to lead to bacteruria, symptomatic UTI, or death than the use of indwelling catheters. This was especially apparent in men without dementia, and the patients overwhelmingly preferred the condom catheters [40].

  – Intermittent catheterization for the following subgroups (Category II)

  - Spinal cord injury patient
  - Patients with bladder emptying dysfunction. This should include postoperative patients, including women with surgery on the genitourinary tract. Hakvoort et al randomized 87 patients who had recent vaginal prolapse surgery and a post void residual > 150 ccs after first void to either foley placement or clean intermittent catheterization (CIC). They found a significant decrease in bacteruria in the CIC group (12 vs 34%). The CIC patients also noted decreased time until return of spontaneous voiding: 18 hours in the CIC group versus 72 hours in the foley group [41]. Moreover, a subsequent study by this same group surveyed the study patients and found that the great majority preferred CIC instead of placement of a foley [42].
  - Children with neurogenic badders, (e.g. myelomeningocele)

– Further research needed on (Unresolved issue)

  - Benefits of urethral stent as an alternative to indwelling catheter in selected patients with bladder outlet obstruction
  - Benefits of suprapubic catheters as an alternative to indwelling urethral catheters in patients requiring short or long term catheterization.

There are studies that have compared suprapubic catheters with urethral catheters. In the gynecology literature, there are few studies. A recent meta-analysis by Healy et al found only 12 randomized controlled trials. They found that although suprapubic catheters had lower overall infection rates when compared to urethral Foleys, (20% compared with 31%), the complication rates were higher (29 % vs 11%) [43]. One study randomized a group of 257 women who underwent anterior repairs with or without vaginal hysterectomy to 3 day suprapubic vs 3 day urethral foley vs 1 day urethral foley. There were fewer infections in the suprapubic group but a significantly higher risk of complications which led to early withdrawal of this arm of the study. Complications included blockage most commonly, urinary retention, and one pyelectasia. They authors concluded that in their trial, the optimal bladder catheter after anterior colporrhaphy was an urethral catheter for 24 hours [44]. Katsumi et al found that men with spinal cord injuries who need chronic catheterization have similar complication rates in terms of UTI, and recurrent bladder and renal calculi with urinary catheters as with suprapubic catheters. Catheter complications rates were similar, though differing in type. Men with urinary catheters had more urethral and scrotal complications, while men with suprapubic tubes had more leakage and 13% required revision [45].

5. Catheter insertion techniques

- Indwelling urethral catheters should be inserted with proper sterile technique and sterile equipment by trained personnel (Category IB)

http://dx.doi.org/10.5772/56709

– Use appropriate hand hygiene before and after insertion or any manipulation of catheter or site (Category 1B)

– Properly secure catheters after insertion to prevent movement and urethral trauma and traction (Category IB)

– Use a closed drainage system (Category IB)

– Use the smallest bore catheter possible to minimize trauma to the urethra and bladder neck (Category II)

- Intermittent catheter recommendations

  – Clean (non-sterile) technique is acceptable for patients requiring chronic intermittent catheterization (CIC) (Category IA)

  – Perform at regular intervals to prevent bladder overdistension (Category IB)

  – Optimal cleaning and storage methods for catheters used for CIC is not determined. (Unresolved issue)

6. Catheter maintenance techniques

- Maintenance of catheter once inserted (all Category IB)

  – Maintain closed drainage system

  – Keep urine flow unobstructed:

  - Avoid kinking
  - Keep collecting bag below level of bladder at all times
  - Empty the collecting bag regularly and avoid contact of the drainage spigot with the collecting container

- Changing of indwelling catheters or drainage bags at fixed intervals is not recommended. Change is only recommended for infection, obstruction of compromise of the system (Category II)
- Do **NOT** use systemic antibiotics routinely for the prevention of CAUTI in patients requiring either short or long term catheterization (Category IB)

  – Further research is needed on the prophylactic use of urinary antiseptics such as methenamine (unresolved issue).

- Do **NOT** use antiseptic solutions to clean the periurethral area while the catheter is in place. Routine hygiene (e.g., cleaning the meatal surface during daily bathing/showering) is appropriate (Category IB)

- Do **NOT** irrigate the catheter unless obstruction is anticipated, such as after prostate or bladder surgery where blood and debris is present within the system. If this is necessary, use closed continuous irrigation. (all Category II)

  – Routine irrigation of bladder with antibiotics is not recommended

  – Routine instillation of antiseptic or antimicrobial solutions into the urinary drainage bag is not recommended

  – Further research is needed on the use of bacterial interference (bladder inoculation with a nonpathogenic bacterial strain) to prevent UTI in patients requiring long term urinary catheterization (Unresolved issue)

- **Catheter materials:** there are antimicrobial catheters available that are coated with silver alloy or antibiotics and may reduce or delay the onset of bacteruria. This is an unresolved issue, but the CDC does recommend consideration of these catheters if the CAUTI rate is not decreasing in an institution despite the implementation of a comprehensive preventive strategy. (Category IB)

  – Silicone catheters might reduce the risk of encrustation in long-term catheterized patients with frequent obstruction (Category II)

  – Hydrophilic catheters, (catheters designed to be lubricated when moistened with water, which eases friction on the urethra upon insertion) might be preferable to standard catheters for patients using CIC (Category II)

  – The benefit of catheter valves in reducing the risk of CAUTI is unclear and further research is needed (unresolved issue). Catheter valves (see Figure 1) are small tubes usually 8 to 12 cm in length with a stopcock mechanism that fit on the end of a foley catheter, replacing the drainage bag. This allows the patient to self empty the catheter in a typical voiding fashion at regular intervals, doing away with the need for a drainage bag. They should not be used by patients with detrusor instability, as bladder wall contractions against a closed bladder outlet could lead to reflux. They also cannot be used by patients with cognitive impairment or limited manual dexterity

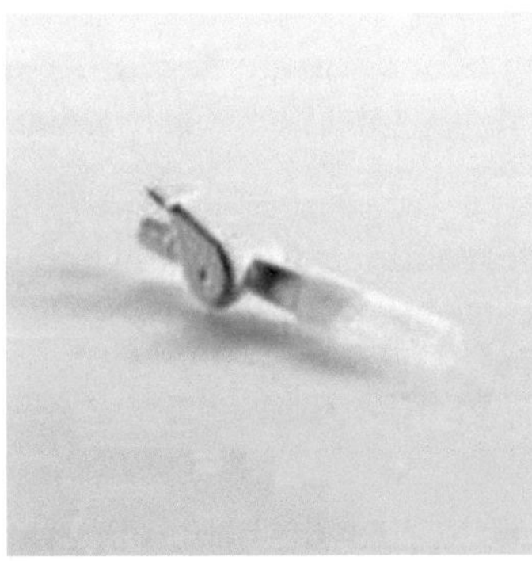

Figure 1. Colpoplast catheter valve

- **Management of obstruction: if this occurs and it is likely that the catheter material is contributing to obstruction, change the catheter (Category IB)**

  – Unresolved issues:

  - Benefit of irrigating catheter with acidifying solutions or use of oral urease inhibitors in patients with long -term indwelling catheters and frequent obstructions.

  - Use of portable bladder scanners to evaluate for obstruction in patients with indwelling catheters and low urine output

  - Use of methenamine to prevent encrustation in patients at high risk for obstruction

- **Specimen collection: (both Category IB)**

  – For culture: obtain these aseptically by aspirating the urine from the needleless sampling port with a sterile syringe after cleaning the port with disinfectant

  – Large volumes or urine for analysis (not culture) can be obtained aseptically from the drainage bag.

7. Quality Improvement (QI) programs

When implemented, there is good evidence that these programs can reduce the risk of CAUTI. (Category IB). Their purpose should be:

- To assure appropriate use of catheters

- To identify and remove catheters that are no longer needed: Alerts or reminders within the medical record that identify patients with catheters in place and note how many days they have been in have been shown to increase the removal rate of catheters. Even placing a sticker on the patient's chart reminding physicians to discontinue unnecessary foleys is beneficial. This simple intervention in a community hospital caused a significant reduction in the rate of CA-UTI after 3 months (7.02 vs 2.08; $P < .001$) and 6 months post-intervention (7.02 vs 2.72; $P < .001$) [46].

- To ensure adherence to hand hygiene and proper care of catheters.

- Guidelines for peri-operative catheter management:

  - Procedure specific guidelines for catheter placement preoperatively and post-operative removal

  - Protocols for management of postoperative urinary retention, such as nurse directed use of intermittent catheterization and use of ultrasound bladder scanners.

8. Other preventive measures

The use of prophylaxis for CAUTI with cranberry products is mentioned in the IDSA guidelines but not in the CDC, with the note that cranberry products should not be used routinely to reduce CAUTI in patients with neurogenic bladders with chronic intermittent OR indwelling catheters. They also noted insufficient date to recommend using cranberry products for other groups. However, these guidelines were published in 2009 before more recent studies that have shown some benefit to cranberry products. The previously cited study by Mutlu, although small, concluded that cranberry capsules could be an encouraging option for the prevention of recurrent UTI in children with neurogenic bladder caused by myelomeningocele who required chronic intermittent catheterization [47.] Because cranberry capsules are safe, inexpensive, well tolerated and don't cause any drug resistance, it would seem worthwhile to use them in these high risk populations as a first line preventive measures.

9. Conclusion

Urinary tract infection is one of the most common healthcare problems facing women, and almost half of women will have a UTI during their lifetime. The incidence is much lower in men, but increases with age. About 15% of women will have problems with recurrent UTI despite having no anatomic abnormalities of the urinary tract. This is likely due to genetic variations in their mucosal protective defense mechanisms that predispose them to bacterial colonization. Preventive strategies should be used liberally in this group of patients and should focus on non-pharmacologic measures first to avoid the ever-increasing drug resistance that is developing worldwide.

Simple hygienic measures are helpful, including proper wiping techniques and voiding after intercourse, and possibly avoiding tub baths. Diaphragms and contraceptive methods containing nonoxynol-9 should be avoided. Cranberry juice or tablets are likely an effective and risk free preventive measure, and should be taken three times daily. Methenamine is an old measure that has been shown to be effective for uncomplicated patients as well. After menopause, these women should use vaginal estrogen therapy which has been shown to decrease recurrences in several studies. If patients continue to have frequent infections despite these measures, a regimen of antibiotic prophylaxis should be started. This can be a single dose taken after intercourse if the patient is sexually active and intercourse triggers an infection. For women who don't have this problem but still have frequent infections, patient- initiated therapy is very effective. The patient has a supply of antibiotic on hand to take at the first sign of symptoms. Finally, for women who continue to have infections despite these strategies, a daily dose of suppression may be needed for 3 to 6 months. However, her risk of infection returns to baseline and remains high when this therapy is discontinued. The antibiotics used most often in suppressive regimens are nitrofurantoin and TMP/SMX

CAUTI remains the leading cause of hospital acquired infections worldwide. Although use of a urethral catheter is at times a necessary part of caring for patients, there are proven steps that can decrease the infection rate. Most importantly, catheters should be placed only for accepted indications and not for incontinence or convenience. For postoperative female patients undergoing uncomplicated procedures, including gynecologic procedures, we should rethink the practice of routine foley placement during the procedure. Instead, consider intermittent in/out catheterization until she is able to ambulate and void satisfactorily. For men without cognitive impairment and obstruction, a condom catheter should be used. More research is needed in the bladder management of the postoperative patient, as well as the role of cranberry to prevent CAUTI. When Foleys are placed, the need for ongoing catheterization should be assessed daily and the catheter discontinued as soon as possible. Reminder systems, whether an electronic reminder or a paper sticker for those not yet using electronic systems, have been shown to lower infection rates and should always be used when a foley is placed.

Author details

Leslie Kammire

Wake Forest School of Medicine, Department of Obstetrics and Gynecology, Winston-Salem, North Carolina, USA

References

[1] Boscia JA, Abrutyn E, Kaye D. Asymptomatic bacteruria in elderly persons: Treat or do not treat?, Ann Intern Med 1987: 106(5) 764-766

[2] World Health Organization, Department of Communicable Disease. Surveillance and Response 2002.

[3] Griebling TL. J Urol 2005; 173(4) 1281-7

[4] Mabeck CE: Treatment of uncomplicated urinary tract infection in non-pregnant women. Postgrad Med J 1972; 48 69-75.

[5] Foxman, B, Chi JW. Health behavior and urinary tract infection in college aged women. J Clin Epidemiol.1990;43(4) 329-37.

[6] Rinke C. Hot Tub Hygiene. JAMA 1983;250(15) 2031-2031.

[7] Dallosso H, McGrother C, Matthews R, Donaldson M, and the Leicestershire MRC Incontinence study group. The association of diet and other lifestyle factors with overactive bladder and stress incontinence: a longitudinal study in women. BJU Int 2003;92 69–77

[8] Arya LA, Myers DL, Jackson ND. Dietary caffeine intake and the risk for detrusor instability: a case-control study. Obstet Gynecol 2000;96 85–9.

[9] Lohsiriwat S, Hirunsai M, Chaiyaprasithi B. Effect of caffeine on bladder function in patients with overactive bladder symptoms. Urol Ann 2011;3 14–8.

[10] Vessey, MP, Metcalfe MA, Mcpherson K, Yeates D. Urinary tract infection in relation to diaphragm use and obesity. Int J Epidemiol 1987 Sep;16(3) 441-4.

[11] Fihn SD, Latham RH, Roberts P et al. Association between diaphragm use and urinary tract infection. JAMA 1985 254(2) 240-5.

[12] Fihn SD, Boyko EJ, Normand EH et al. Association between use of spermicide-coated condoms and Escherichia coli urinary tract infection in young women. Am J Epidemiol 1996 ;144(5) 512-20.

[13] Stamm WE, Raz R. Factors contributing to susceptibility of postmenopausal women to recurrent urinary tract infections. Clin Infect Dis 1999;28 723–725.

[14] Bergman J, Schjøtt J, Blix HS. Prevention of urinary tract infections in nursing homes: lack of evidence-based prescription? BMC Geratr 2011;11 69.

[15] Lavigne JP, Bourg G, Combescure Cet al. In-vitro and in-vivo evidence of dose-dependent decrease of uropathogenic Escherichia coli virulence after consumption of commercial Vaccinium macrocarpon (cranberry) capsules. Clin Microbiol Infect 2008 ;(4) 350-5.

[16] Wang CH, Fang CC, Chen NC et al.. Cranberry-Containing Products for Prevention of Urinary Tract Infections in Susceptible Populations: A Systematic Review and Meta-analysis of Randomized Controlled Trials. Arch Intern Med 2012;172(13) 988-96.

[17] Stapleton AE, Dziura J, Hooton TM et al. Recurrent Urinary Tract Infection and Urinary E. coli in women ingesting cranberry juice daily: a randomized controlled trial. Mayo Clin Proc 2012;87(2) 143-150.

[18] Salo J, Uhari M, Helminen M, et al. Cranberry juice for the prevention of recurrences of urinary tract infection in children: a randomized placebo-controlled trial. Clin Infect Dis 2012;54(3) 340-6.

[19] Mutlu H, Ekinci Z. Urinary Tract Infection Prophylaxis in Children with Neurogenic Bladder with Cranberry Capsules: Randomized Controlled Trial. ISRN Pediatr 2012;2012 317280.

[20] Wing DA, Rumney PJ, Preslicka CW, Chung JH. Daily cranberry juice for the prevention of asymptomatic bacteriuria in pregnancy: a randomized, controlled pilot study. J Urol 2008;180(4) 1367-1372.

[21] Lavigne et al. BMC Res Notes 2011;4 522.

[22] Efros M, Bromberg W, Cossu L et al. Novel concentrated cranberry liquid blend, UTI-STAT with Proantinox, might help prevent recurrent urinary tract infections in women. Urology 2010 Oct;76(4) 841-5.

[23] Wing DA, Rumney PJ, Preslicka CW, Chung JH. Daily cranberry juice for the prevention of asymptomatic bacteriuria in pregnancy: a randomized, controlled pilot study. J Urol 2008;180(4) 1367-1372.

[24] Wang CH, Fang CC, Chen NC et al.. Cranberry-Containing Products for Prevention of Urinary Tract Infections in Susceptible Populations: A Systematic Review and Meta-analysis of Randomized Controlled Trials. Arch Intern Med 2012;172(13) 988-96.

[25] Lorenzo-Gómez MF, Padilla-Fernández B, García-Criado FJ, Mirón-Canelo JA, Gil-Vicente A, Nieto-Huertos A, Silva-Abuin JM. Int Urogynecol J 2013 Jan;24(1) 127-34.

[26] Lee BB, Simpson JM, Craig JC, Bhuta T. Methenamine hippurate for preventing urinary tract infections. Cochrane Database Syst Rev 2007 Oct 17;(4) CD003265.

[27] Gupta et al. Patient Initiated treatment of uncomplicated recurrent urinary tract infections in young women. Ann Intern Med 2001;135(1) 9-16.

[28] Zhong YH, Fang Y, Zhou JZ et al. Effectiveness and safety of patient initiated single-dose versus continuous low-dose antibiotic prophylaxis for recurrent urinary tract infections in postmenopausal women: a randomized controlled study. J Int Med Res 2011;39(6) 2335-43.

[29] D'Arcy PF. Nitrofurantoin. Drug Intell Clin Pharm 1985;19 540-6.

[30] Rudenko N, Dorofeyev A. Prevention of recurrent lower urinary tract infections by long-term administration of fosfomycin trometamol. Double blind, randomized, parallel group, placebo controlled study. Arzneimittelforschung 2005;55(7) 420-7.

[31] Naber KG, et al. Surveillance study in Europe and Brazil on clinical aspects and antimicrobial resistance epidemiology in females with cystitis (ARSEC): implications for empiric therapy. Eur Urol 2008;54 1164-78.

[32] The Direct Medical Costs of Healthcare-Associated Infections in U.S. Hospitals and the Benefits of Prevention. CDC publication 2009.

[33] Smith PW, Bennett G, Bradley S et al. American Journal of Infection Control 2008;36(7) 504–535.

[34] R.J. Pratt, C.M. Pellowe, J.A. Wilson, H.P. Loveday, PJ. Harper, S.R.L.J. Jones *et al.* EPIC 2: national evidence-based guidelines for preventing healthcare-associated infections in NHS hospitals in England J Hosp Infect 65 (Suppl. 1) (2007), pp S1-S64.

[35] European and Asian guidelines on management and prevention of catheter-associated urinary tract infections. Int J Antimicrob Agents 31 (Suppl. 1) (2008), pp. S68–S78.

[36] Center for Disease Control. Healthcare Infection Control Practice Advisory Committee. *Guidelines for Prevention of Catheter-Associated Urinary Tract Infections* 2009.

[37] Hooton TM, Bradley SF, Cardenas DD et al. Diagnosis, Prevention, and Treatment of Cather-Associated Urinary Tract Infection in Adults: 2009 International Clinical Prac-

tice Guidelines from the Infectious Disease Society of America. Clinical infectious Disease 2010;50 625-663

[38] Conway LJ, Larson EL. Guidelines to prevent catheter-associated urinary tract infection: 1980 to 2010 Heart & Lung: The Journal of Acute and Critical Care. 2012;41(3) 271-83.

[39] Center for Disease Control. Healthcare Infection Control Practice Advisory Committee. *Guidelines for Prevention of Catheter-Associated Urinary Tract Infections* 2009.

[40] [40] J Saint S, Kaufman SR, Rogers MA, Baker PD, Ossenkop K, Lipsky BA. Condom vs Indwelling urinary catheters: a randomized controlled trial. Am Geriatr Soc 2006;54(7) 1055-61.

[41] [41] Hakvoort RA, Thijs SD, Bouwmeester FW, Broekman AM, Ruhe IM, Vernooij MM, Burger MP, Emanuel MH, Roovers JP. Comparing clean intermittent catheterisation and transurethral indwelling catheterisation for incomplete voiding after vaginal prolapse surgery: a multicentre randomised trial. BJOG. 2011;118(9) 1055-60.

[42] Hakvoort RA, Nieuwkerk PT, Burger MP, Emanuel MH, Roovers JP. Patient preferences for clean intermittent catheterisation and transurethral indwelling catheterisation for treatment of abnormal post-void residual bladder volume after vaginal prolapse surgery. BJOG.2011;118(11) 1324-8.

[43] Healy EF, Walsh CA, Cotter AM, Walsh SR. Suprapubic compared with transurethral bladder catheterization for gynecologic surgery: a systematic review nad metanalsyis. Obstet Gynecol 2012;120(3) 678-87.

[44] Kringel U, Reimer T, Tomczak S, Green S, Kundt G, Gerber B. Postoperative infections due to bladder catheters after anterior colporrhaphy: a prospective, randomized three-arm study. Int Urogynecol J 2010 ;21(12) 1499-504.

[45] Katsumi HK, Kalisvaarti, JF, Ronningen LD, Hovey RM. Urethral versus suprapubic catheter: chooseing the best bladder management for male spinal cord injury patients with indwelling catheters. Spinal Cord 2010;(48) 325-329.

[46] Bruminhent J, Keegan M, Lakhani A, Roberts IM, Passalacqua J. Effectiveness of a simple intervention for preventin of catheter-associated urinary tract infections in a community teaching hospital. Am J Infect Control 2010;38(9) 689-93.

[47] Mutlu H, Ekinci Z. Urinary Tract Infection Prophylaxis in Children with Neurogenic Bladder with Cranberry Capsules: Randomized Controlled Trial. ISRN Pediatr. 2012;2012:317280. doi: 10.5402/2012/317280. Epub 2012 Jul 1

Chapter 2

Prevention of Catheter-Associated Urinary Tract Infections

Ioannis Efthimiou and Kostadinos Skrepetis

Additional information is available at the end of the chapter

http://dx.doi.org/10.5772/52957

1. Introduction

Urinary catheter placement is an extremely common medical intervention. It can be used either temporarily, for example to drain a full bladder, to monitor urine output or it can be indwelling for long term drainage. While urinary catheters are a safe medical practice, complications can and do arise from their use and can be a source of morbidity for hospital or nursing home residents. The term "catheter fever" was used for the first time in 1883 [1] and it has been 50 years since Beeson, et al., recognized the potential harms arising from urethral catheterization and penned an editorial to the American Journal of Medicine titled "The case against the catheter" [2]. Nowadays, it is well recognized that catheter-associated infections (CAUTIs) cause the vast majority of nosocomial urinary tract infections (UTIs) [3, 4]. Designing an effective strategy for prevention of CAUTI presupposes an in depth knowledge of epidemiology, pathogenesis, microbiology and risk factors for all medical personnel.

2. Epidemiology

Generally, UTIs comprise the 40% of hospital-acquired infections [5-9] and 80% of them are CAUTIs [10-11]. CAUTIs are directly related with the use of indwelling urinary catheters [12, 13]. Up to 25% of patients have an indwelling catheter placed at some time during their hospital stay [3]. CAUTIs are associated with increased morbidity, mortality, length of hospital stay and cost. It has been estimated that one episode of nosocomial acquired UTI adds 1–3 days of extra hospital stay [3]. Moreover, the annual cost of CAUTIs is estimated to be $340-370 million [14, 15].

The prevalence of nosocomial-acquired UTIs in Urology departments was estimated to be 10% in the Pan European Prevalence study and 14% in the Pan Euro Asian Prevalence study [16]. In the same study, the largest group was that of asymptomatic bacteriuria (29%) followed by cystitis (26%), pyelonephritis (21%), and urosepsis (12%). There were 0.61 catheters per patient. 51% of the catheters were transurethral with continuous drainage, 10% transurethral with open drainage, 2% clean intermittent catheterization, 11% suprapubic catheters, 12% nephrostomy tubes and 14% ureteral stents [16].

Urinary catheters are responsible for nearly 97% of UTIs in ICUs [12, 13]. Recently published data, regarding device-associated infections within intensive care units (ICUs) collected by hospitals participating in the International Nosocomial Infection Control Consortium (INICC) between January 2003 and December 2008, showed an overall mean CAUTIs rate from 0.4 to 13.9 per 1000 urinary catheter-days [17]. The distribution was lower in the surgical-cardio-thoracic ICUs and higher in the Neurosurgical ICUs. Mean crude mortality and mean excess mortality rate for CAUTIs in ICUs were 32.9% and 18.5% respectively. Surgical-cardiothoracic and Neurosurgical ICUs had the highest urinary catheter utilization ratios (0.93 and 0.86 respectively). Pediatric ICUs had the lowest mean CAUTI and mean catheter utilization ratios (4.4 and 0.17 respectively) [17].

It has also been reported that 7.5% and 5.4% of nursing home residents in the USA and Europe respectively are long-term catheterized [18, 19]. Indwelling catheters in nursing home residents are used more commonly in men than in women with the most common indication that of urinary retention in men (87%) and in women (58%) [20]. In a web-based survey among nursing home residents, the percentage of residents with indwelling/suprapubic catheters and infections was 21.7% [21]. The overall incidence and prevalence of symptomatic UTs in the studied population were 29.2% and 1.64% respectively.

3. Pathogenesis-mechanisms

The main route of infection in CAUTI is ascending. This happens by two main mechanisms: Firstly, extraluminally through migration of bacteria along catheter surfaces and secondly due to colonization of the catheter bag or contamination of the junction between the catheter and the catheter bag [22, 23].

In an animal model, it was found that in short-term catheterization, less than 7 days, contamination of the drainage spout or accidental disconnection of the drainage tube resulted in bacteriuria within a short time (32-48 hours). If a strict sterile closed drainage system was maintained, the extraluminal route assumed more importance in the development of bacteriuria; however this pathway was considerably slower (72-168 hours) [22].

In a prospective clinical study, 66% of the infections were extraluminally acquired and 34% were derived from intraluminal contaminants [23]. Gram-positive cocci and yeasts were more likely to be extraluminally acquired than were gram-negative bacilli, which caused CAUTIs by both routes equally. In the same study, there were no significant differences in pathogenetic mechanisms between the two sexes.

http://dx.doi.org/10.5772/52957

Origination of bacteria is from endogenous organisms either from rectum or colonizing the patient's perineum [23-25]. In one of these studies, colonization of periurethral area was more prevalent in women than in men [23].

Bacteria adhere to catheters via a variety of molecules such are fibriae, heamagglutinin or capsular polysaccharide [26]. Once bacteria have attached to surfaces of catheters, they grow in glycocalyx-enclosed microcolonies and produce a biofilm on the catheter surface which is associated with CAUTIs [27]. Studies have shown that bacteria in this microenvironment are resistant to antibiotics for two reasons [28-30]. Firstly, they are metabolically inactive, perhaps due to low concentration of oxygen [28] and secondly, biofilm acts as a physical barrier to diffusion of antibiotics and host defense mechanisms [29-31]. On the contrary, planktonic-free floating bacteria in urine are susceptible to antibiotics [32-33]. It is worth noting that these two populations are not always identical.

Indwelling catheters not only act as a nidus for bacteria but they also cause physical trauma to normal urothelium, they may promote inflammatory reaction, alter metabolic activity and cell proliferation which facilitates bacterial infection [26]. Recently, an in vitro study which used bladder cancer cell cultures found that catheters are involved in disruption of bladder epithelial cell membranes as a result of physical abrasion which was followed by delayed inflammation in response to bacterial infection [34].

Figure 1 presents schematically all the possible mechanisms involved in pathogenesis of CAUTIs.

4. Microbiology of CAUTIs

The majority of uropathogens are fecal contaminants or skin residents from the patient's own native or transitory microflora that colonize the periurethral area. As it has already been mentioned CAUTIs caused by gram-positive cocci and yeasts are far more likely to be extraluminally acquired than were gram-negative bacilli, which caused CAUTIs by both routes equally [23].

CAUTIs in short-term catheterization is usually produced by single species and *Escherichia coli* remains the most common infecting organism. However, a wide variety of other gram negative microorganisms may be isolated like *Klebsiela* spp., *Enterobacter* spp, and *Serratia* spp [35, 36]. Gram positive cocci including coagulase-negative staphylococci and *Enterococcus* spp have also been isolated [37, 38]. Other species commonly found in patients with short-term catheterization are *Proteus* spp. and *Morganella morganii* [37]. *Proteus mirabilis* is isolated more frequently than *E. coli* in men. Anaerobic organisms also contribute to infection [39]. Colonization with methicillin-resistant *S. aureus* (MRSA) occurs frequently in institutions with endemic MRSA [40, 41]. Although initially biofilms contain single species of microbes, they progressively become polimicrobic, especially in long term-catheterization [39].

P.aurignosa, enterococci and *Candida* spp. are more commonly found in ICUs [17, 42]. *Providencia stuartii* has been isolated in nursing home residents as a result of cross infection [43].

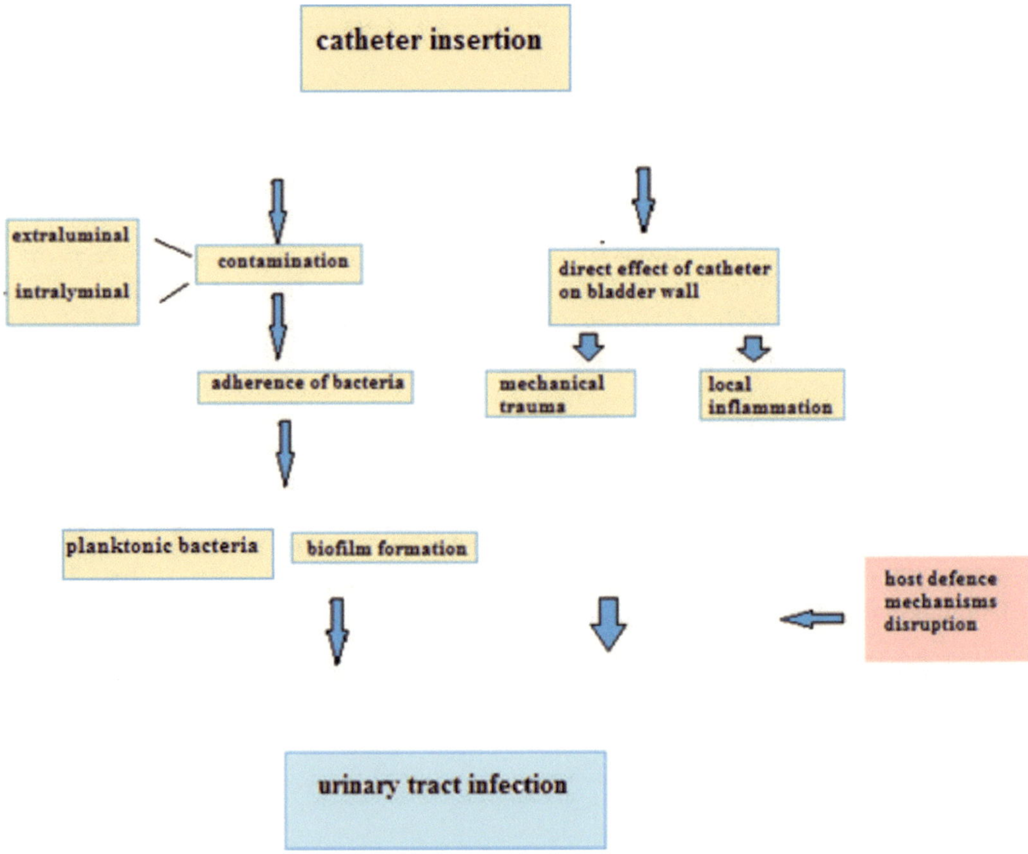

Figure 1. Pathogenesis of CAUTIs.

For some species of bacteria, it has been shown that the longer an indwelling catheter is in place, the grater the concentration of bacteria in urine. This number decreases when the catheter is replaced by a new one [44]. In particular, higher concentration was observed before catheter replacement for species such are *P. mirabilis, P. stuartii, M. morganii, P. aeruginosa,*and enterococci, whereas concentrations of *E. coli* and *K. pneumoniae* were similar in the 2 specimens [44].

Patients with blocked catheters are also more often colonized with *Proteus mirabilis* and *Providencia stuartii* than are patients without blocked catheters [45].

5. Risk factors War

Warren found that patients with indwelling bladder catheters had a 3% to 10% incidence of bacteria growth per day with development of bactiuria in most within one month [46]. Several prospective clinical studies have evaluated the risk factors for development of nosocomial UTI, catheter acquired bacteriuria and CAUTI [47-52]. All the risk factors are presented in table 1.

Catheter-related	**Patient-related**	**Enviroment/Personnel-related**
Duration of cateterization [48-50]	Female [47, 48, 50]	Hospitalization in Orthopeadic department [49]
Lack of urimeter drainage [48]	Elderly [47]	Hospitalization in Urology department [49]
Colonization of drainage bag [48]	Critical ill [47]	Insertion after the 6th day of hospitalization [49]
Reason for catheterization [48]	Diabetes mellitus [48]	Catheterization outside the operating theatre [49]
Breaks in closed system [47]	Renal failure (Cr>2mg/dl) [48]	Lack of antibiotics (only for the first 4 days of catheterization) [47-50]
	Periurethral colonization [53]	Improper care [47, 49]

Table 1. Risks factors for development of CAUTI.

Many of these factors have been evaluated in more than one clinical trial. The duration of catheterization is the most important risk factor. The daily risk for acquiring bacteriuria was higher among patients ultimately catheterized for greater than or equal to 7 days than among those ultimately catheterized for less than 7 days [49]. Systematic antibiotic use exerts a protective use only for short-term catheterization (16% versus 32%) but has not been proven of value for long–term drainage [47-50].

Also increased risk has been found among women. This is probably due to their anatomy, causing an easier access of the perineal flora to the bladder along the catheter as it traverses the shorter female urethra and absence of prostatic secretions. Diabetic patients have susceptibility in acquiring urinary infection, probably due to increased prevalence of perineal colonization by potential pathogens, and increased ability of the urine of some diabetics to support microbial growth. Chronic renal failure is another risk factor for the development of urinary infections as a result of metabolic disorders which promote in secondary disorders of all components of immunity [54].

Finally, critically ill patients (uremic encephalopathy, viral encephalitis, bacterial peritonitis, diabetic ketoacidosis, stroke, and alcoholic liver disease with septicemia) are more susceptible to UTIs especially to candidal UTIs [55].

6. Prevention and control of CAUTIs

6.1. Indications for Indwelling catheter insertion

Selection of patients for catheterization should be standardized and reserved for certain medical conditions. Appropriate indications for the use of catheters are acute urinary retention for temporary relief of anatomical (e.g. BPH, urethral stricture) or functional obstruction (e.g. neurogenic bladder), perioperative in select procedures (e.g. after major surgical procedures or cases performed under spinal anesthesia), and the frequent, accurate measurement of urine output in critically ill patients e.g. hemodynamic unstable [55-64].

Other appropriate uses are for patient's comfort at the end of life, patients who are incontinent and there is a risk of contamination with sacral, perineal wound or buttock trauma, and prolonged immobilization under conditions such as unstable spine or pelvic fracture [57-64].

The catheter should remain in place only as long as the reason for insertion is still present. For example, postoperatively as a patient has been mobilized, the catheter is no longer necessary to remain. Clinicians should avoid use of indwelling catheters for management of convenience of personnel and urine measurement [55, 63-64]. Urine output monitoring in oliguric patients is not an indication for indwelling catheter. It can be measured, using either bladder scanner or condom catheters [65]. Urine residual can be estimated with a bladder scanner as well. Patients with BPH and bladder outlet obstruction, who are not candidates for definite surgical procedure, can be managed effectively with minimal invasive techniques e.g. bladder neck incision, prostatic stent placement [66].

6.2. Right catheter practice

Aseptic catheter insertion remains one of the cornerstones in preventing CAUTI. Initially, perform hand hygiene immediately before and after insertion or any manipulation of the catheter device or site. Ensure that only properly trained persons (eg, hospital personnel, family members, or patients themselves) familiar with proper aseptic catheter insertion and maintenance are given this responsibility. In the acute care hospital setting, insert the smallest urinary catheter whenever possible, using aseptic technique and sterile equipment. Smaller catheters (14 French or 16 French) and 10-ml balloons should be utilized, as larger catheters have been shown to be a risk factor for the development of UTI [56]. These larger catheters tend to increase the amount of residual urine that can lead to the reinoculation of the bladder and increase the risk of blockage of the periurethral glands that leads to UTI, urethral irritation, and erosion. Instead large-bore catheters are appropriate for short-term practice e.g. management of heamaturia, postoperatively after urologic procedures.

Sterile equipment includes necessary for catheterization: sterile gloves, disposable fenestrated drape, sponges, an appropriate antiseptic or sterile solution for periurethral cleaning, and a single-use packet of lubricant jelly for insertion. After insertion secure the catheter to prevent movement and urethral traction and keep the urine bag below the level of the bladder with a urine bag hanger [67].

It is important to remember that hands are colonized by resident and transient bacteria and for this reason they should be cleaned before and after every patient contact and before an aseptic technique is carried out, even when sterile gloves are also used [68].

It is not necessary to use an antiseptic preparation to clean the urethral meatus before catheter insertion However, to avoid contamination of the sterile procedure field, it is advisable to use a sterile solution to cleanse the urethral meatus. Sterile saline or water may be considered [69].

An appropriate lubricant from a single-use container should be used during catheterization to minimize trauma and infection [70]. A number of studies considered the use of lubricants in urological procedures, concluding that the vulnerable urothelium can only be protected by an unbroken film of lubricant [71]. The method of dipping the catheter tip in the lubricant gel does not meet the requirement to coat the urethra and should be discouraged [70, 71]. The lubricant can be wiped off at the entry to the urethra and, therefore, will not reach the narrow more vulnerable parts. The urethra is not dilated by the insertion of a lubricating gel, allow for the comfortable passage of the catheter. There is potential for infection because of contamination of the container from repeated use.

Wherever the procedure is performed, especially in nurse home residents, hazardous waste, wet or soiled dressings and soiled incontinence pads must be removed from the immediate area. In some cases, general cleaning may be required to ensure that there is an appropriate area in which to establish the sterile field [72].

6.3. Special types of catheters

Latex and polytetrafluoroethylene-coated are appropriate for short-term drainage instead of silicon and hydrogel-coated which are appropriate for long term use. Collectively, these data are presented on table 2 [73]. Studies have shown that gram negative bacteria adhere less to siliconized rubber than to other catheter materials [74]. Proteus mirabilis have showed the greatest adherence from the gram-negative bacteria and like most bacteria has the most marked adherence to the red rubber catheter [75]. They can be used to reduce the risk of encrustation in long-term catheterized patients who have frequent obstruction [64].

Bacterial adherence is even more decreased in hydrophilic catheter surface and this effect is more pronounced for enteroccoci [76]. Hydrophilic catheters might be preferable to standard catheters for patients requiring intermittent catheterization [63, 64].

<table>
<tr><th>Catheter material</th><th>Length of use</th></tr>
<tr><td>Latex or plastic</td><td>Short term (up to 14 days)</td></tr>
<tr><td>Polytetrafluoroethylene-coated latex</td><td>Short term (up to 28 days)</td></tr>
<tr><td>All silicone</td><td rowspan="4">Long term (up to 12 weeks)</td></tr>
<tr><td>Silicone elastomer-coated latex</td></tr>
<tr><td>Hydrogel-coated latex</td></tr>
<tr><td>Hydrogel-coated silicone</td></tr>
</table>

Table 2. Different types of catheters [73].

In a recent meta analysis, Schumm et al concluded that silver oxide catheters were not associated with a statistically significant reduction in bacteriuria in short-term catheterized hospitalized adults [76]. Instead, silver alloy catheters (silver-latex-hydrogel) were found to significantly reduce at least a half the incidence of asymptomatic bacteriuria in hospitalized adults catheterized for <1 week in comparison to standard catheters. At >1 week of catheterization the estimated effect was smaller but still less in the silver alloy group [77]. Also, it has been shown that hydrogel coated and silver-hydrogel-latex catheters had little difference in bacterial adherence [76].

According to above findings and considering the extra cost of silver alloy catheters of 80%-130% compared to standard ones [79], most of the guidelines do not recommend their use in standard practice [78].

Antibiotic-coated catheters were also developed in an effort to prevent or delay the onset of catheter-associated bactiuria. Nitrofurazone impregnated catheters has been more detailed studied in antibiotic trials and they suggest benefit in terms of a decreased risk of asymptomatic bactiuria during the first week [77]. Initially, nitrofurazone diffuses from the catheter surface producing inhibition zones but this effect is progressively lost and bacteria attach and proliferate due to concentration reduction [76]. Overall antibiotic impregnated catheters regardless of antibiotic type reduce bactiuria in hospitalized adults who are catheterized for < 1 week however further research is needed on this field [77].

6.4. Closed drain systems

All guidelines advised on maintaining a closed sterile drainage system (figure 2) for indwelling catheters [78]. Also, the three most recent guidelines recommend the use of preconnected catheter and drainage system with sealed junctions [78]. If breaks in aseptic technique, disconnection, or leakage occur, replace the catheter and collecting system using aseptic technique and sterile equipment [63, 64].

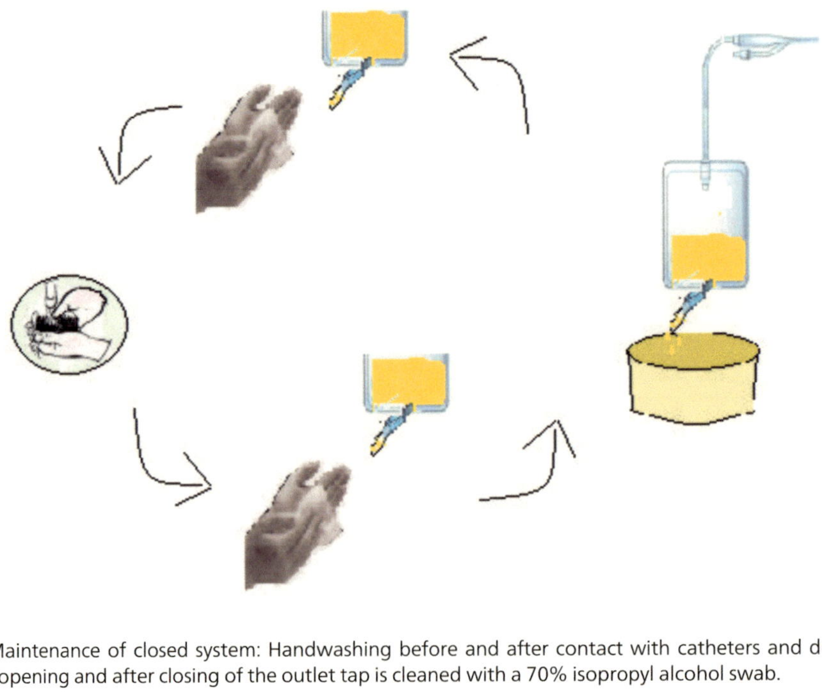

Figure 2. Maintenance of closed system: Handwashing before and after contact with catheters and drainage bags and before opening and after closing of the outlet tap is cleaned with a 70% isopropyl alcohol swab.

6.5. Alternative techniques of urine drainage

Alternative methods of catheterization that potentially reduce the risk of CAUTIs, including condom and suprapubic catheters and intermittent catheterization are available. Condom catheters, while useful for male patients with functional disabilities such as restricted mobility or dementia plus incontinence, who lack bladder outlet obstruction, require meticulous care to avoid complications such is skin maceration [80, 56]. They are ideal for nighttime use and are more comfortable, less painful, and less restrictive than indwelling catheters [81]. The condom catheter must be changed every day. In a descriptive point-prevalence survey in hospitalized patients the risk of UTI was higher in those wearing condom catheters than in those with a chronic indwelling catheter [82]. In contrast, in another study in home nursing home residents, the incidence of UTI was lower in men wearing external condom catheters than in men with indwelling catheters [83]. Randomized control studies are required to clarify further this field. Condom catheters may be preferable for incontinent men who will not manipulate their catheter frequently [84].

According to IDSA guidelines, suprapubic catheterization may be considered as an alternative to short-term indwelling urethral catheterization to reduce catheter associated bacteriuria [63]. In a meta analysis, comparing transurethral and suprapubic catheter for short-term use found that the latter one had reduced microbiologic morbidity [85]. However, data are insufficient to make a recommendation as to whether suprapubic catheterization is preferable to long-term indwelling urethral catheterization for reduction of catheter associated-bacteriuria or CAUTI [63]. Advantages of suprapubic route are: comfort and less local complications such as meatal erosion, prostatitis and epididymitis [85, 86].

Intermittent catheterization is the preferred method of catheterization in patients who have bladder dysfunction, specifically neurogenic bladder. Common causes of neurogenic bladder are spinal cord injury and myelomeningocele. Intermittent catheterization should be considered an alternative to short-term or long-term indwelling urethral catheterization to reduce catheter associated-bacteriuria and an alternative to short-term or long-term indwelling urethral catheterization to reduce CAUTI. Data are insufficient to make a recommendation as to whether intermittent catheterization is preferable to suprapubic catheterization for reduction of catheter associated bacteriuria or CAUTI [63].

6.6. Chemoprophylaxis

Most experts do not recommend routinely using prophylactic antibiotics for catheterized patients because of their cost, potential adverse effects and role in encouraging antibiotic drug resistance [87-89]. Prophylactic antibiotic drug therapy may be appropriate for those who require relatively short-term, 3-14 days, catheterization and are at high risk for complications from a UTI [24, 89]. In a recent double-blind, placebo-control randomized trial a single dose of prophylaxis did not affect the rate of bacteriuria and UTI 14 days after the catheter removal [90]. Thus, prophylaxis might not be needed for routine removal of urinary catheters in otherwise healthy non-genitourinary surgical patients postoperatively. However, this rule does not apply to individuals undergoing surgery of the urinary tract, where factors such as intact urothelium, antegrade flow, foreign bodies and urine pH may all be altered and correspondingly require antimicrobial use around the time of catheter removal [91].

If bacteriuria occurs prior to removal of the catheter, the patient should be treated with appropriate antimicrobial therapy. Urinalysis or urine cultures should be obtained following removal of the catheter to assure sterility of the urinary tract. [89]. Prophylaxis with trimethoprim-sulphamethoxazole should be given to patients undergoing renal transplantation and requiring catheterization. Also data from randomized control trials suggest that systemic antibiotic prophylaxis is justified for transurethral resection of prostate in men with an indwelling catheter or bacteriuria before surgery [92, 93].

For those requiring long-term catheterization prophylactic antibiotics only postpone at best bacteriuria [84].

6.7. Intravesical instillation of prophylactic factors

Antibiotic and antiseptic solution instillation either continuously of intermittently has been studied in the past for prevention of CAUTIs [94, 95]. Although bladder irrigation with topical antimicrobial agents (e.g. neomycin, polymyxin B) have demonstrated some value in preventing UTI when an open drainage system was used, little overall benefit has been seen with closed systems. So in view of the potential for local toxic effects and the complexity of this method, antibacterial irrigation currently cannot be recommended [84].

6.8. Prevention of CAUTIs in general surgery

The urinary bladder is routinely catheterized during major surgery to monitor urine output throughout the perioperative period and to avoid the risk for urinary retention and bladder over distension. Traditionally, the catheter is inserted in the patients' bladder at the beginning of surgery and stays for a few days according to postoperative course and local policy.

It is also common practice to catheterize the bladder in those surgical patients receiving epidural analgesia and to leave the catheter in situ as long as epidural analgesia is maintained due to high rate of postoperative urinary retention (24%) [96, 97]. When local anesthetics are injected in the epidural space act on the sacral and lumbar nerve fibers in the spinal cord, blocking the transmission of afferent and efferent nervous impulses from and to the bladder. This results in decreased sensation of urgency and impaired bladder detrusor contraction.

Late studies on these target groups encourage early catheter removal [98, 99]. These studies have shown that early removal of the catheter was not associated with a higher incidence of recatheterization and UTIs, implying that catheter can safely be removed on the first postoperative day [98]. Leaving the bladder catheter as long as the epidural analgesia is maintained results in a higher incidence of UTI and prolonged hospital stay [99].

Early removal of urinary catheters is a part of modern postoperative management named by many authors as "fast-track surgery" and has truly reduced the rate of UTIs from 24% to 4% [100]. As it has already been mentioned, routine antibiotic prophylaxis might not be needed for removal of urinary catheters in non-urological surgical patients postoperatively with intact urothelium [90].

6.9. Prevention of CAUTIs in neurogenic bladder

Intermittent catheterization is one of the most effective and commonly used methods of bladder management in patients with a neurogenic bladder. Regular bladder emptying reduces intravesical bladder pressure and improves blood circulation in the bladder wall, making the bladder mucous membrane more resistant to infectious bacteria (figure 3) [101]. So inserting the catheter several times during the day, episodes of bladder over distention are avoided.

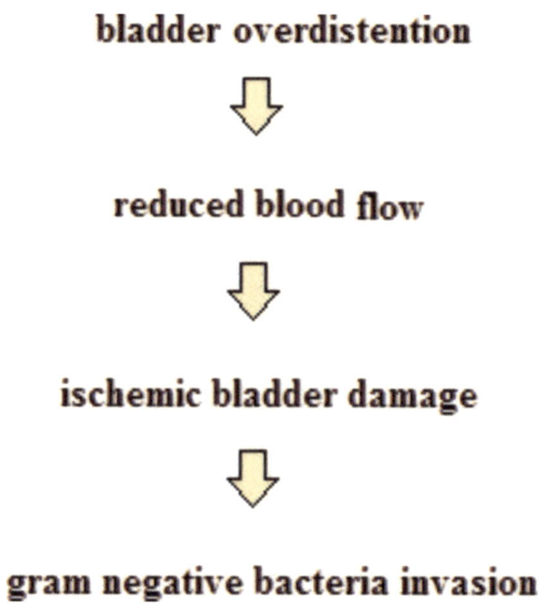

Figure 3. Pathogenesis of UTIs in patients with neurogenic bladder according to Lapides et al theory [101].

Measures that decrease the incidence of UTIs in patients with neurogenic bladder are: Adherence to strict basic daily protocol with solid education and understanding about intermittent catheterization technique helps and avoids most of UTIs in this category of patients [102, 103]. It was also been proven that catheterization between at least four times for most individuals helps them to maintain a mean volume of catheterization of less than 400ml and reduces the incidence of UTIs [104].

According to Cochrane Review Database, there are no definitive studies showing the incidence of UTIs is improved with any catheter technique, type, or strategy [105]. Regarding the use of cranberry, there is limited evidence from clinical trials that suggests that they don't seem to be effective in preventing or treating UTIs in spinal cord population [106].

6.10. Prevention of CAUTIs in elderly with long-term catheter

Elderly are prone to long-term catheterization for many reasons and many of them are either surgically correctable e.g. a large symptomatic cystocele in women can easily be corrected with pelvic floor reconstruction or medically associated e.g. due to antihistamines, anticholinergics or tricyclic antidepressants and may be managed with medication discontinuation or treatment modification.

Long-term catheters are almost always associated with bacteriuria [107]. Strategy for prevention in these cases includes [108]: Hydration in order to promote washout of bacteria and maintain proper function of catheter. Routine catheter exchange e.g. every 4-6 weeks, depending on each patient. Patients with tendency to catheter encrustation require more frequent catheter exchange. Routine antibiotic prophylaxis is not required as it has already mentioned above it inevitably leads to development of drug resistant bacteria [87, 88, 89].

6.11. Local policy development for reduction of CAUTIs

Development of a local strategy from hospitals may contribute in reduction in the incidence of CAUTIs. The components of this policy are presented on table 3 [109].

Periodic training in aseptic technique, maintenance and removal
Education about CAUTIs and alternatives to indwelling catheter
Implement a system for documenting: indications for catheter insertion, date and time of catheter insertion, individual who performed insertion, date and time of catheter insertion, date and time of catheter removal
Use of standardized methodology for performing CAUTI surveillance
Family and caregiver teaching, discharge instructions
Use of removal triggers
Early catheter removal program

Table 3. Components of a local policy in reduction of CAUTIs [109].

Most of them have been evaluated in a number of studies and have shown their effectiveness in reduction of CAUTIs. For example, the utility of various reminder systems, physical or virtual, has been examined in a number studies with encouraging results [110-116]. In one study paper based prewritten 'stop orders' or protocols and stickers to encourage clinicians to insert catheters only when absolutely necessary and remove as soon as no longer proved useful in reduction of CAUTIs [110]. Bruminhent et al. [111] found that placing reminder stickers on patient medical records significantly reduced the rate of CAUTIs (7.02 vs. 2.08, P<0.001) after 3 months. This study was also associated with lower antibiotics costs and no impact on overall mortality. Another study by Loeb et al. [114] randomized 692 patients with indwelling catheters to usual care vs. prewritten orders for catheter removal if specified criteria are not present. This study reported a significant reduction of duration of inappropriate urinary catheterization in hospitalized patients but did not reduce urinary tract infections. Virtual reminders involve the use of electronic devices to remind nurses and clinicians about catheter removal [117]. Automatic stop orders can be tied to computerized catheter orders or reminders can be sent via pagers [115]. However, these systems contribute to higher costs as they involve more time and manpower resources. A systemic review by Blodgett [116] found three trials on virtual reminders that were associated with reduction in the rates of CAUTI, duration of catheterization and overall costs.

7. Conclusion

Prevention is the main step against CAUTI. Priorities with proven value are the appropriate use and early removal of catheters, aseptic insertion, the maintenance of a closed urinary drainage system and implement of a structured local policy. However, there are still many challenges that need more clarification from research and well designed randomized control trials.

Author details

Ioannis Efthimiou[1] and Kostadinos Skrepetis[2]

1 Department of Urology, University Hospital of Alexandroupolis, Greece

2 Department of Urology, General Hospital of Kalamata, Greece

References

[1] Clark, A. Remarks on catheter fever. Lancet (1883). ii:1075–1077.

[2] Beeson, P. B. The case against the catheter. Am J Med (1958).

[3] Haley, R, Culver, D, White, J, Morgan, W. M, & Emori, T. G. The nationwide nosocomial infection rate: A new need for vital statistics. Am J Epidemiol (1985).

[4] Danchaivijitr, S, Dhiraputa, C, Cherdrungsi, R, Jintanothaitavorn, D, & Srihapol, N. Catheter-associated urinary tract infection. J Med Assoc Thai (2005). Suppl 10) 26–30.

[5] Maki, D. G, & Tambyah, P. A. Engineering out the risk for infection with urinary catheters. Emerg Infect Dis (2001). , 7(2), 342-7.

[6] Wagenlehner, F. M, Loibl, E, Vogel, H, & Naber, K. G. Incidence of nosocomial urinary tract infections on a surgical intensive care unit and implications for management. Int J Antimicrob Agents (2006). Suppl 1) S, 86-90.

[7] Girard, R, Mazoyer, M. A, Plauchu, M. M, & Rode, G. High prevalence of nosocomial infections in rehabilitation units accounted for by urinary tract infections in patients with spinal cord injury. J Hosp Infect (2006). , 62(4), 473-9.

[8] Vonberg, R. P, Behnke, M, Geffers, C, Sohr, D, Ruden, H, Detternkofer, M, et al. Device-associated infection rates for non-intensive care unit patients. Infect Control Hosp Epidemiol (2006). , 27(4), 357-61.

[9] Wald, H. L, & Kramer, A. M. Nonpayment for harms resulting from medical care: catheter-associated urinary tract infections. JAMA (2007). , 298(23), 2782-4.

[10] Anderson, D. J, Kirkland, K. B, Kaye, K. S, Thacker, P. A, Kanafani, Z. A, & Auten, G. Underresourced hospital infection control and prevention programs: penny wise, pound foolish? Infect Control Hosp Epidemiol (2007). , 28(7), 767-73.

[11] Willson, M, Wilde, M, Webb, M. L, Thompson, D, Parker, D, Harwood, J, et al. Nursing interventions to reduce the risk of catheter-associated urinary tract infection: part 2: staff education, monitoring, and care techniques. J Wound Ostomy Continence Nurs (2009). , 36(2), 137-54.

[12] Richards, M. J, Edwards, J. R, Culver, D. H, & Gaynes, R. P. Nosocomial infections in combined medical-surgical intensive care units in the United States. Infect Control Hosp Epidemiol (2000). , 21(8), 510-515.

[13] Krieger, J. N, Kaiser, D. L, & Wenzel, R. P. Nosocomial urinary tract infections: secular trends, treatment and economics in a university hospital. J Urol (1983). , 130(1), 102-106.

[14] Klevens, R. M, Edwards, J. R, Richards, C. L, et al. Estimating healthcare-associated infections and deaths in U.S hospitals, 2002. Public Health Rep (2007). , 122(2), 160-166.

[15] United States Department of Health and Human ServicesAction plan to prevent healthcare-associated infections (2009). http://http://www.premierinc.com/safety/topics/HAI.accessed 12 June 2012).

[16] Bjerklund Johansen TECek M, Naber K, Stratchounski L, Svendsen MV, Tenke P; PEP and PEAP study investigators; European Society of Infections in Urology. Prevalence of hospital-acquired urinary tract infections in urology departments. Eur Urol. (2007). , 51(4), 1100-11.

[17] Rosenthal, V. D, Maki, D. G, Jamulitrat, S, Medeiros, E. A, Todi, S. K, Gomez, D. Y, et al. INICC Members. International Nosocomial Infection Control Consortium (INICC) report, data summary for 2003-2008, issued June (2009). Am J Infect Control. 2010; e2., 38(2), 95-104.

[18] Warren, J. W, & Steinberg, L. Hebel RJ & Tenney J H. The prevalence of urethral catheterization in Maryland nursing homes. Archives of Internal Medicine, (1989). , 149(7), 1535-1537.

[19] Sørbye, L. W, Finne-soveri, H, Ljunggren, G, Topinková, E, & Bernabei, R. Indwelling catheter use in home care: elderly, aged 65+, in 11 different countries in Europe. Age and Ageing, (2005). , 34(4), 377-381.

[20] Jonsson, K, Loft, E-S. o. n, Nasic, A. L, & Hedelin, S. H. A prospective registration of catheter life and catheter interventions in patients with long-term indwelling urinary catheters. Scand J Urol Nephrol. (2011). , 45(6), 401-5.

[21] Tsan, L, Davis, C, Langberg, R, Hojlo, C, Pierce, J, Miller, M, et al. Prevalence of nursing home-associated infections in the Department of Veterans Affairs nursing home care units. Am J Infect Control. (2008). , 36(3), 173-9.

[22] Nickel, J. C, Grant, S. K, & Costerton, J. W. Catheter-associated bacteriuria. An experimental study. Urology. (1984). , 26(4), 369-75.

[23] Tambyah, P. A, Halvorson, K. T, & Maki, D. G. A prospective study of pathogenesis of catheter-associated urinary tract infections. Mayo Clin Proc. (1999). , 74(2), 131-6.

[24] Stamm, W. E. Catheter-associated urinary tract infections: epidemiology, pathogenesis, and prevention. Am J Med. (1991). B) 65S-71S.

[25] Daifuku, R, & Stamm, W. E. Association of rectal and urethral colonization with urinary tract infection in patients with indwelling catheters. JAMA. (1984). , 252(15), 2028-30.

[26] Barford, J, & Coates, A. The pathogenesis of catheter-associated urinary tract infection. J of Inf Prev (2009). , 10(2), 50-56.

[27] Nickel, J. C, Downey, J. A, & Costerton, J. W. Ultrastructural study of microbiologic colonization of urinary catheters. Urology. (1989). , 34(5), 284-91.

[28] Elves, A. W, & Feneley, R. C. Long-term urethral catheterization and the urine-biomaterial interface. Br J Urol (1997). , 80(1), 1-5.

[29] Nickel, J. C, Costerton, J. W, Mclean, R. J, & Olson, M. Bacterial biofilms: influence on the pathogenesis, diagnosis and treatment of urinary tract infections. J Antimicrob Chemother (1994). Suppl. A) , 31-41.

[30] Nickel, J. C, Gristina, P, & Costerton, J. W. Electron microscopic study of an infected Foley catheter. Can J Surg (1985). , 28(1), 50-1.

[31] Nickel, J. C, Ruseska, I, Wright, J. B, & Costerton, J. W. Tobramycin resistance of Pseudomonas aeruginosa cells growing as a biofilm on urinary catheter material. Antimicrob Agents Chemother (1985). , 27(4), 619-24.

[32] Olson, M. E, Nickel, J. C, Khoury, A. E, Morck, D. W, Cleeland, R, & Costerton, J. W. Amdinocillin treatment of catheter-associated bacteriuria in rabbits. J Infect Dis (1989). , 159(6), 1065-72.

[33] Kunin, C. M, & Steele, C. Culture of the surfaces of urinary catheters to sample urethral flora and study the effect of antimicrobial therapy. J Clin Microbiol (1985). , 21(6), 902-8.

[34] Barford, J. M, Hu, Y, Anson, K, & Coates, A. R. A biphasic response from bladder epithelial cells induced by catheter material and bacteria: an in vitro study of the pathophysiology of catheter related urinary tract infection. J Urol. (2008). , 180(4), 1522-6.

[35] Warren, J. W. Catheter-associated urinary tract infection. Infect Dis Clin North Am (1997).

[36] Cadedda, G, Fioravanti, P, Gasparini, P. M, & Gaetti, R. Etiologic, prognostic and social health aspects of urinary infections in hospitalized elderly with an indwelling urinary catheter. Minerva Urol Nefrol (1997).

[37] Nicolle, L. E. Catheter-related urinary tract infection. Drugs Aging (2005). , 22(8), 627-639.

[38] Gross, P. A, Harkavy, L. M, Barden, G. E, & Flower, M. F. The epidemiology of nosocomial enterococcal urinary tract infection. Am J Med Sci. (1976). , 272(1), 75-81.

[39] Alling, B, Brandberg, A, Seeberg, S, & Svanborg, A. Aerobic and anaerobic microbial flora in the urinary tract of geriatric patients during long-term care. J Infect Dis. (1973). , 127(1), 34-9.

[40] Bradley, S. F, Terpenning, M. S, Ramsey, M. A, et al. Methicillin- resistant Staphylococcus aureus: colonization and infection in a long-term care facility. Ann. Intern. Med. (1991). , 115(6), 417-422.

[41] Strausbaugh, C, Jacobson, C, Sewell, L, Potter, S, & Ward, T. Methicillin-resistant Staphylococcus aureus in extended care facilities: experiences in a Veteran's Affairs Nursing Home and a review of the literature. Infect. Control Hosp. Epidemiol. (1991). , 12(1), 36-45.

[42] Bougnoux, M. E, Kac, G, Aegerter, P, Enfert, d, & Fagon, C. JY; CandiRea Study Group. Candidemia and candiduria in critically ill patients admitted to intensive care units in France: incidence, molecular diversity, management and outcome. Intensive Care Med. (2008). , 34(2), 292-9.

[43] Nicolle, L, Bjornson, J, & Harding, G. MacDonell J. Bacteriuria in elderly institutionalized men. N. Engl. J. Med. (1983). , 309(23), 1420-1425.

[44] Tenney, J. H, & Warren, J. W. Bacteriuria in women with long-term catheters: paired comparison of indwelling and replacement catheters. J Infect Dis (1988). , 157(1), 199-202.

[45] Kunin, C. M. Blockage of urinary catheters: role of microorganisms and constituents of the urine on formation of encrustations. J Clin Epidemiol (1989). , 42(9), 835-42.

[46] Waren, J. W. Catheter associated bacteria in long-term facilities. Infect Control Hosp Epidemiol (1994). , 15(8), 557-62.

[47] Garibaldi, R. A, Burke, J. P, Dickman, M. L, & Smith, C. B. Factors predisposing to bacteriuria during indwelling urethral catheterization. N Engl J Med. (1974). , 291(5), 215-9.

[48] Platt, R, Polk, B. F, Murdock, B, & Rosner, B. Risk factors for nosocomial urinary tract infection. Am J Epidemiol. (1986). , 124(6), 977-85.

[49] Shapiro, M, Simchen, E, Izraeli, S, & Sacks, T. G. A multivariate analysis of risk factors for acquiring bacteriuria in patients with indwelling urinary catheters for longer than 24 hours. Infect Control. (1984). , 5(11), 525-32.

[50] Johnson, J. R, Roberts, P. L, Olsen, R. J, Moyer, K. A, & Stamm, W. E. Prevention of catheter-associated urinary tract infection with a silver oxide-coated urinary catheter: clinical and microbiologic correlates. J Infect Dis. (1990). , 162(5), 1145-50.

[51] Riley, D. K, Classen, D. C, Stevens, L. E, & Burke, J. P. A large randomized clinical trial of a silver-impregnated urinary catheter: lack of efficacy and staphylococcal super infection. Am J Med. (1995). , 98(4), 349-56.

[52] Huth, T. S, Burke, J. P, Larsen, R. A, Classen, D. C, & Stevens, L. E. Clinical trial of junction seals for the prevention of urinary catheter-associated bacteriuria. Arch Intern Med. (1992). , 152(4), 807-12.

[53] Bryan, C. S, & Reynolds, K. L. Hospital-acquired bacteremic urinary tract infection: epidemiology and outcome. J Urol (1984). , 132(3), 494-498.

[54] Vaziri, N. D, Pahl, M. V, Crum, A, & Norris, K. Effect of uremia on structure and function of immune system. J Ren Nutr. (2012). , 22(1), 149-56.

[55] Kamat, U. S, Fereirra, A, Amonkar, D, Motghare, D. D, & Kulkarni, M. S. Epidemiology of hospital acquired urinary tract infections in a medical college hospital in Goa. Indian J Urol (2009). , 25(1), 76-80.

[56] Wong, E. S. Guideline for prevention of catheter associated urinary tract infections. Am J Infect Control (1983). , 11(1), 28-36.

[57] Pratt, R. J, Pellowe, C. M, Wilson, J. A, Loveday, H. P, Harper, P. J, et al. EPIC 2: national evidence-based guidelines for preventing healthcare associated infections in NHS hospitals in England. J Hosp Infect (2007). Suppl. 1) S, 1-64.

[58] Tenke, P, & Kovacs, B. Bjerklund Johansen TE, T. Matsumoto, Tambyah PA, Naber KG. European and Asian guidelines on management and prevention of catheter-associated urinary tract infections. Int J Antimicrob Agents (2008). Suppl. 1) S, 68-78.

[59] Lo, E, Nicolle, L, Classen, D, Arias, K. M, Podgorny, K, Anderson, D. J, et al. Strategies to prevent catheter associated urinary tract infections in acute care hospitals. Infect Control Hosp Epidemiol (2008). Suppl. 1) S, 41-50.

[60] Parker, D, Callan, L, Harwood, J, Thompson, D. L, Wilde, M, & Gray, M. Nursing interventions to reduce the risk of catheter-associated urinary tract infection. Part 1: catheter selection. J Wound Ostomy Continence Nurs (2009). , 36(2), 23-34.

[61] Willson, M, Wilde, M, Webb, M-L, Thompson, D, Parker, D, Harwood, J, et al. Nursing interventions to reduce the risk of catheter-associated urinary tract infection: part 2: staff education, monitoring, and care techniques. J Wound Ostomy Continence Nurs (2009). , 36(2), 137-54.

[62] Parker, D, Callan, L, Harwood, J, Thompson, D, Webb, M-L, Wilde, M, et al. Catheter-associated urinary tract infections: fact sheet. J Wound Ostomy Continence Nurs (2009). , 36(2), 156-9.

[63] Hooton, T. M, Bradley, S. F, Cardenas, D. D, Colgan, R, Geerlings, S. E, Rice, J. C, et al. Diagnosis, prevention, and treatment of catheter-associated urinary tract infection in adults: 2009 international clinical practice guidelines from the Infectious Diseases Society of America. Clin Infect Dis (2010). , 50(5), 625-63.

[64] Gould, C. V, Umscheid, C. A, Agarwal, R. K, Kuntz, G, & Pegues, D. A. Healthcare Infection Control Practices Advisory Committee. Guideline for prevention of catheter-associated urinary tract infections 2009. Infect Control Hosp Epidemiol (2010). , 31(4), 319-26.

[65] Kunin, C. M. Nosocomial urinary tract infections and the indwelling catheter: What is new and what is true? Chest (2001). , 120(1), 10-12.

[66] Perry, M. J, Roodhouse, A. J, Gidlow, A. B, Spicer, T. G, & Ellis, B. W. Thermo-expandable intraprostatic stents in bladder outlet obstruction: an 8-year study. BJU Int. (2002). , 90(3), 216-23.

[67] AnonymousEvaluation of aseptic techniques and chlorhexidine on the rate of catheter associated urinary-tract infection. Southampton Infection Control Team. Lancet (1982). , 1(8263), 89-91.

[68] Pratt, R. J, Pellowe, C, Loveday, H. P, Robinson, N, Smith, G. W, Barrett, S, et al. The EPIC Project: developing national evidence-based guidelines for preventing healthcare associated infections. Phase I: guidelines for preventing hospital-acquired infections. Department of Health (England). J Hosp Infect (2001). Suppl.) S, 3-82.

[69] Webster, J, Hood, R. H, Burridge, C. A, Doidge, M. L, Phillips, K. M, & George, N. Water or antiseptic for periurethral cleaning before urinary catheterization: A randomized controlled trial. Am J Infect Control (2001). , 29(6), 389-394.

[70] National Institute for Clinical Excellence ((2003). Infection Control: Prevention of Healthcare associated Infection in Primary and Community CareNICE, London.

[71] Sperling, H, Lümmen, G, & Rübben, H. Use of lubricants in urology. Indications and results. Urologe A. (2005). , 44(6), 662-6.

[72] Magnall, J, & Watterson, L. Principles of aseptic technique in urinary catheterization. Nurs Stand. (2006). , 21(8), 49-56.

[73] Bardsley, A. Use of lubricant gels in urinary catheterization. Nurs Stand. (2005). , 20, 41-6.

[74] Sugarman, B. Adherence of bacteria to urinary catheters. Urol Res. (1982). , 10(1), 37-40.

[75] Roberts, J. A, Fussell, E. N, & Kaack, M. B. Bacterial adherence to urethral catheters. J Urol. (1990). Pt 1) 264-9.

[76] Desai, D. G, Liao, K. S, Cevallos, M. E, & Trautner, B. W. Silver or nitrofurazone impregnation of urinary catheters has a minimal effect on uropathogen adherence. J Urol. (2010). , 184(6), 2565-71.

[77] Schumm, K, & Lam, T. B. Types of urethral catheters for management of short-term voiding problems in hospitalized adults: a short version Cochrane review. Neurourol Urodyn. (2008). , 27(8), 738-46.

[78] Conway, L. J, & Larson, E. L. Guidelines to prevent catheter-associated urinary tract infection: 1980 to 2010. Heart Lung. (2012). , 41(3), 271-83.

[79] Johnson, J. R, Kuskowski, M. A, & Wilt, T. J. Systematic review: antimicrobial urinary catheters to prevent catheter-associated urinary tract infection in hospitalized patients. Ann Intern Med. (2006). , 144(2), 116-26.

[80] Hirsh, D. D, Fainstein, V, & Musher, D. M. Do condom catheter collecting systems cause urinary tract infection? JAMA (1979). , 242(4), 340-341.

[81] Ouslander, J. G, & Greengold, B. Chen S: Complications of chronic indwelling urinary catheters among male nursing home patients: A prospective study. J Urol (1987). , 138(5), 1191-1195.

[82] Zimakoff, J, Stickler, D. J, Pontoppidan, B, et al. Bladder management and urinary tract infections in Danish hospitals, nursing homes, and home care: a national prevalence study. Infect Control Hosp Epidemiol (1996). , 17(4), 215-221.

[83] Ouslander, J. G, Greengold, B, & Chen, S. External catheter use and urinary tract infections among incontinent male nursing home patients. J Am Geriatr Soc. (1987). , 35(12), 1063-70.

[84] Saint, S, & Lipsky, B. A. Preventing catheter-related bacteriuria: should we? Can we? How? Arch Intern Med. (1999). , 159(8), 800-8.

[85] Mcphail, M. J, Abu-hilal, M, & Johnson, C. D. A meta-analysis comparing suprapubic and transurethral catheterization for bladder drainage after abdominal surgery. Br J Surg. (2006). , 93(9), 1038-44.

[86] Chenoweth, C. E. Infections Associated with Urinary Catheters. Catheter-Related Infections. In: Seifert H, Jansen B, Farr BM (Eds). Catheter-related infections. Merkell Decker New York; (2006). , 490-518.

[87] Meares EM JrCurrent patterns in nosocomial urinary tract infections. Urology. (1991). Suppl 3) 9-12.

[88] Platt, R, Polk, B. F, Murdock, B, & Rosner, B. Prevention of catheter-associated urinary tract infection: a cost-benefit analysis. Infect Control Hosp Epidemiol. (1989). , 10(2), 60-4.

[89] Schaeffer, A. J. Catheter-associated bacteriuria. Urol Clin North Am. (1986). , 13(4), 735-47.

[90] Van Hees, B. C, Vijverberg, P. L, Hoorntje, L. E, Wiltink, E. H, Go, P. M, & Tersmette, M. Single-dose antibiotic prophylaxis for urinary catheter removal does not reduce the risk of urinary tract infection in surgical patients: a randomized double-blind placebo-controlled trial. Clin Microbiol Infect. (2011). , 17(7), 1091-4.

[91] Schaeffer, E. M. Re: Single-dose antibiotic prophylaxis for urinary catheter removal does not reduce the risk of urinary tract infection in surgical patients: a randomized double-blind placebo-controlled trial. J Urol. (2012).

[92] Amin, M. Antibacterial prophylaxis in urology: a review. Am J Med. (1992). A) 114S-117S.

[93] Qiang, W, & Jianchen, W. MacDonald R, Monga M, Wilt TJ. Antibiotic prophylaxis for transurethral prostatic resection in men with preoperative urine containing less than 100,000 bacteria per ml: a systematic review. J Urol. (2005). , 173(4), 1175-81.

[94] Gelman, M. L. Antibiotic irrigation and catheter-associated urinary tract infections. Nephron. (1980).

[95] Warren, J. W, Platt, R, Thomas, R. J, Rosner, B, & Kass, E. H. Antibiotic irrigation and catheter-associated urinary-tract infections. N Engl J Med. (1978). , 299(11), 570-3.

[96] Baldini, G, Bagry, H, Aprikian, A, & Carli, F. Postoperative urinary retention: anesthetic and perioperative considerations. Anesthesiology. (2009). , 110(5), 1139-1157.

[97] Kemp, D, & Tabaka, N. Postoperative urinary retention: part IIVa retrospective study. J Post Anesth Nurs. (1990). , 5(6), 397-400.

[98] Zaouter, C, Kaneva, P, & Carli, F. Less urinary tract infection by earlier removal of bladder catheter in surgical patients receiving thoracic epidural analgesia. Reg Anesth Pain Med. (2009). , 34(6), 542-8.

[99] Basse, L, Werner, M, & Kehlet, H. Is urinary drainage necessary during continuous epidural analgesia after colonic resection? Reg Anesth Pain Med. (2000). , 25(5), 498-501.

[100] Zargar-shoshtari, K, Connolly, A. B, Israel, L. H, & Hill, A. G. Fast-track surgery may reduce complications following major colonic surgery. Dis Colon Rectum. (2008). , 51(11), 1633-40.

[101] Lapides, J, Diokno, A. C, Silber, S. M, & Lowe, B. S. Clean, intermittent self-catheterization in the treatment of urinary tract disease. 1972. J Urol. (2002). , 167(4), 1584-6.

[102] Cardenas, D. D, & Hoffman, J. M. Hydrophilic catheters versus noncoated catheters for reducing the incidence of urinary tract infections: A randomized controlled trial. Archives of Physical Medicine & Rehabilitation, (2009). , 90(10), 1668-1671.

[103] Wyndaele, J. J. Complications of intermittent catheterization: Their prevention and treatment. Spinal Cord, (2002). , 40(10), 536-541.

[104] Bakke, A, Digranes, A, & Høisaeter, P. A. Physical predictors of infection in patients treated with clean intermittent catheterization: a prospective 7-year study. Br J Urol. (1997). , 79(1), 85-90.

[105] Moore, K. N, Fader, M, & Getliffe, K. Long-term bladder management by intermittent catheterization in adults and children. Cochrane Database Syst Rev. (2007). CD006008.

[106] Jepson, R. G, & Craig, J. C. Cranberries for preventing urinary tract infections. Cochrane Database Syst Rev. (2008). CD001321.

[107] Tambyah, P. A, & Maki, D. G. Catheter-associated urinary tract infection is rarely symptomatic: a prospective study of 1,497 catheterized patients. Arch Intern Med (2000). , 160(5), 678-682.

[108] Wagenlehner, F. M, Cek, M, Naber, K. G, Kiyota, H, & Bjerklund-johansen, T. E. Epidemiology, treatment and prevention of healthcare-associated urinary tract infections. World J Urol. (2012). , 30(1), 59-67.

[109] Fink, R, Gilmartin, H, Richard, A, Capezuti, E, Boltz, M, & Wald, H. Indwelling urinary catheter management and catheter-associated urinary tract infection prevention practices in Nurses Improving Care for Healthsystem Elders hospitals. Am J Infect Control. (2012). Epub ahead of print].

[110] Apisarnthanarak, A, Thongphubeth, K, Sirinvaravong, S, et al. Effectiveness of multifaceted hospital wide quality improvement programs featuring an intervention to remove unnecessary urinary catheters at a tertiary care center in Thailand. Infect Control Hosp Epidemiol (2007). , 28(7), 791-798.

[111] Bruminhent, J, Keegan, M, Lakhani, A, et al. Effectiveness of a simple intervention for prevention of catheter-associated urinary tract infections in a community teaching hospital. Am J Infect Control (2010). , 38(9), 689-693.

[112] Gokula, R. M, Smith, M. A, & Hickner, J. A. Emergency room staff education and use of a urinary catheter indication sheet improves appropriate use of Foley catheters. Am J Infect Control (2007). , 35(9), 589-593.

[113] Fakih, M. G, Dueweke, C, Meisner, S, et al. Effect of nurse-led multidisciplinary rounds on reducing the unnecessary use of urinary catheterization in hospitalized patients. Infect Control Hosp Epidemiol (2008). , 29(9), 815-819.

[114] Loeb, M, Hunt, D, & Halloran, O. K, et al. Stop orders to reduce inappropriate urinary catheterization in hospitalized patients: a randomized controlled trial. J Gen Intern Med (2008). , 23(6), 816-820.

[115] Cornia, P. B, Amory, J. K, Fraser, S, et al. Computer-based order entry decreases duration of indwelling urinary catheterization in hospitalized patients. Am J Med (2003). , 114(5), 404-407.

[116] Blodgett, T. J. Reminder systems to reduce the duration of indwelling catheters: a narrative review. Urol Nurs (2009). , 29(5), 369-379.

[117] Tambyah, P. A, & Oon, J. Catheter-associated urinary tract infection. Curr Opin Infect Dis. (2012). , 25(4), 365-70.

Chapter 3

Problem of Catheter Associated Urinary Tract Infections in Sub–Saharan Africa

Mohamed Labib and Nenad Spasojevic

Additional information is available at the end of the chapter

http://dx.doi.org/10.5772/55371

1. Introduction

Ever since the introduction of the first indwelling catheter with an inflated baloon in 1853 by Dr. Jean Francois Reybard, a French Surgeon, it has become clear what a useful instrument Urologists were given, but at the same time over the years of usage it became obvious that the use of such a simple instrument goes along with some risks as well [1].

To this date every day urological practice cannot be imagined without a catheter but at the same time it has became clear that the use of the catheter has inevitably put the Urologist in a position where he has to deal with the complications that arise from catheterization [2].

One of the most common complications of catheterization is catheter-associated urinary tract infection (CAUTI).

Catheter-associated urinary tract infection (CAUTI) is defined as bacteriuria or funguria with a count of more than 10^3 CFUs/ml [2, 4].

Catheter associated urinary tract infection is the most common nosocomial infection in hospitals worldwide and the incidence has been reported to be approximately 35% [2].

In the USA, CAUTI is the most common nosocomial infection, accounting for more than 1 million cases each year in hospitals and nursing homes (Tambyah and Maki 2000) [3].

Duration of catheterization is a significant risk factor for CAUTI.

It is well accepted that bacterial colonisation with catheterisation is inevitable with some reports estimating the risk to be in the region of 5% per day with almost 100% colonisation risk at 7 to 10 days of catheterisation. The incidence of bacteriuria has been estimated to be about 3% to 10% higher each day after catheter insertion [4].

Bacteriuria is therefore almost always present in these patients and, unless symptomatic, does not require treatment. Although most Catheter-associated urinary tract infections are asymptomatic, they often precipitate unnecessary antimicrobial therapy [2, 4].

Although there have been recommendations to treat CAUTIs only when they are symptomatic, the symptoms associated with CAUTI have not been clearly defined. (Tambyah and Maki 2000) [3]

Apart from duration of catheterisation, which is a well established, CAUTI risk factor in settings such as Sub-Saharan Africa (Zambia in this case), there are a few more worth mentioning such as: catheterization in unsterile enviroment, use of unsuitable catheters for long term catheterization (eg. Latex catheters changed on monthly basis), use of homemade drainage systems, diabetes, malnutrition and immunocompromized (HIV) patient catheterization is also of higher risk for CAUTI.

Most CAUTIs are derived from the patient's own colonic flora and the catheter predisposes to UTI in several ways. The most important risk factor for the development of catheter-associated bacteriuria is the duration of catheterization [2].

The best prevention of CAUTIs would be not to use a catheter at all however this, unfortunately, is not likely in the near future, so attention should be focused on two issues in order to reduce catheter-associated urinary tract infections and these are : Catheter system should be closed and Duration of catheterization should be minimal.

By all means medical staff should also consider an alternative to indwelling urethral catheter. In appropriate patients suprapubic catheterization or intermittent catheterization are much better options than indwelling urethral catheterization.

In everyday medical practice, use of urethral catheters in Sub-Saharan Africa (Zambia) is very common. There are several reasons for this practice but the main ones are the shortage of educated and trained staff and inaccessibility of health care facilities.

Having Zambia for example, country area 752 618 km^2, and population of over 12 million at present there are 8 Urologists.

Urologist patient ratio in Zambia is 1:1,500 000 and furthermore 7 out of 8 Urologists are in the largest hospital in the country, University Teaching Hospital in Lusaka which means that there is severe shortage in urological services.

Two of the most common urological conditions in this population are BPH and urethral strictures and these two are associated with catheterization in most cases urethral and less suprapubic catheterization.

In this setting urethral catheterization is well established procedure for relieving bladder outlet obstruction and the patients are usually on the long term catheterization until they are attended by a Urologist. This creates a huge window of opportunity for development of CAUTIs, which is, unfortunately, the case; and moreover, pushing the health system with limited resources to its final limits.

Average time spent on waiting by BPH patient to be attended by a Urologist is approximately 4 months and in addition to this another 3 to 4 months waiting for operation, if there is indicated surgical procedure. Having all this in mind, it is easy to see that the average catheterization time can take months rather than days and that the considerable risk of symptomatic CAUTIs is present.

Catheters are routinely changed on monthly basis and the catheterization in unsterile enviro-ment, the poor quality of the catheters and lack of urine bags are predisposing factors for CAUTIs.

In order to try to prevent CAUTIs in settings like this, patients on the long term urethral catheterization are advised to take care of hygiene (both gentialia and catheter) and to keep well hydrated (bladder wash out).

It is not uncommon that in the case of symptomatic CAUTI simple change of catheter and hydration can do as much as antibiotic treatment especially having in mind limited choice of antibiotics and the fact that most of the bacteria causing CAUTI are multidrug resistant.

In 2005, we did a research of using intermittent catheterization after urethral stricture management and it showed a reduce in the incidence of UTI by 30%. The idea cannot be implemented as standard policy for the patients because of lack of human resources.

The risk of developing a catheter-related UTI rises by 5% for each day the catheter remains in place (Tambyah et al, 2002) [3]. Having this fact in mind it is clear that catheter associated urinary tract infections can hardly be avoided. On the other hand, in some settings like Sub-Saharan Africa (Zambia) the benefit of catheterization is greater than the risk of getting complications related to catheter associated urinary tract infection.

Although it is widely accepted that the short term catheterization (less than 28 days) is preferred to long term catheterization (over 28 days), in our setting, the majority of the catheterized patients are in the group of long term catheterization. This is because of the fact that urological service is almost exclusive to the biggest medical centres in the country whilst almost completely absent in other health care facilities. This means that indication for catheterization and follow up of the catheterized patients is done mainly by many others health care practitioners for quite a long period of time before the patient actually reaches the Urologist.

From experience, a patient booked for urological procedure like transvesical prostatectomy can spend more than five months waiting for the operation and all this time will be catheterized and therefore will be affected with catheter associated urinary tract infection.

Since we unfortunately don't have any research conducted in this way we can only assume that this prolonged catheterization and subsequent CAUTI can have an impact on some patients in terms of prolonged postoperative recovery, wound infection, bladder fistula etc.

However there are certain steps that might be helpful in order to prevent catheter associated urinary tract infections. In our opinion, which is based on practicing Urology in settings like Sub-Saharan Africa (Zambia), these steps are mainly addressing the issues of real need for catheterization, technique of catheterization and last but not least catheter care.

Before every catheterization there are certain standards that need to be met in order to postpone catheter associated urinary tract infection. These are:

- Assessing the need for catheterization
- Appropriate type catheter selection
- Aseptic technique of catheter insertion
- Catheter care

Practicing every day Urology in Sub Saharan Africa (Zambia) brings certain challenges in order to find the balance between patients' needs, available equipment and up to date urological guidelines and these are sometimes extremely difficult to meet.

In African settings it is quite difficult to avoid catheter associated urinary tract infections and this fact is mainly because factors such as:

1. **Assessments of the patient** that may need catheterization is made quite often by nurses and not by doctors and this fact is mainly due to the fact that vast majority of medical facilities are understaffed.

This fact can result not only in catheter associated urinary tract infection but also in unnecessary catheterisation in the first place.

The other issue is availability of the Urologist; seven out of eight Zambian Urologists are placed in the capital, Lusaka, and this is almost the same issue in other Sub-Saharan countries.

It is not uncommon that patients spend months being catheterized before reaching the urologist and starting urological investigations.

2. **Catheter selection** can have an impact on CAUTI.

Nowadays it is a well-documented fact that some of the catheters can actually reduce the incidence of catheter associated urinary tract infections.

Silver-alloy-coated catheters can reduce catheter associated urinary tract infections by up to 45% (Davenport K, KeelyFX –J.Hosp.Infect- 2005)

However in settings like Sub-Saharan Africa (Zambia) the lack of appropriate catheters is more or less the rule.

Furthermore, the quality of catheters available in this part of the world is often poor and this can also result in catheter associated urinary tract infections.

It has been observed that the catheters we are using are prone to encrustation after a short period of time and this can only be an additional factor in promoting the infection.

The most common type of catheter in use in this setting is Latex silicone coated Foley catheter, and when it comes to sizes there is no rule but the most common size is 18 Ch, although it is not uncommon that the patient is catheterized with catheter size 22 Ch, regardless of gender, simply because the fact that this is the only available catheter at the time of catheterization.

The other explanation for usage of the catheters with diameter greater than 18 Ch is belief that these catheters can provide better drainage which can be the true in certain conditions (e.g. haematuria, pyuria) but in most other cases (in our experience) the catheter size 16 Ch will make sufficient urine drainage.

Catheterization of children is even more complicated because of lack of adequate paediatric catheters (most common one is latex silicone coated Foley catheter and most common size available is size 8 Ch).

3. **Catheterization** in Sub-Saharan setting is quite often performed using clean rather than aseptic technique which of course may lead to CAUTI. Main reason for this is that not all of the necessary equipment for catheterization is available all the time especially in remote areas. The things that are available most of the time are: examination gloves, methylated spirit, cotton wool, catheters, and syringes.

Doctors and/or nurses use examination gloves, cotton wool balls and sterile water to clean the genital region, afterwards methylated spirit is used for cleaning and then the catheter is inserted using K-Y gel.

Anaesthetic gels are rarely used for catheterisation because they are not always available and the other reason is the price of these gels (5 US$ per tube which can be more than the daily salary for the majority of the population).

In our practice we usually use catheters sizes 16 Ch and 18 Ch for male catheterization and for female catheterization sizes 14 Ch and 16 Ch, but the actual size that we are going to use is mainly limited with the catheters available.

Although there are certain recommendations to use the smallest possible catheters in order to minimize urethral trauma, pressure necrosis of urethral mucosa and bladder spasms, Urologists in Sub-Saharan Africa are mainly forced to come up with the best possible solution regarding the equipment that is available.

After the catheterization urine bag (if available) is placed and fixed to the patient's leg, it has been observed that patients in our setting are reluctant to have urine bags fixed to the leg, but prefer keeping urine bags in the trouser pockets or even in the inside pocket of the jackets and in this way, make drainage virtually impossible. This is one of the factors that promote catheter associated urinary tract infection due to poor drainage and the urine stasis. Another thing that has been observed is poor urine bag care and this fact also makes the urine bag a source and generator of infection.

Furthermore, the urine bags are not available in remote rural areas and, therefore, it is not unusual to see patient having the same urine bag for months and this fact makes them inadequate to use for the majority of patients.

To avoid urine bags we prefer to use stoppers, this is of course is the case if continuous drainage is not indicated. All the patients, regardless of their education and background, are easily trained to take care of the stopper. The other good thing about the stopper is that in case of unavailability it can be easily substituted with the 2ml syringe plunger which is common

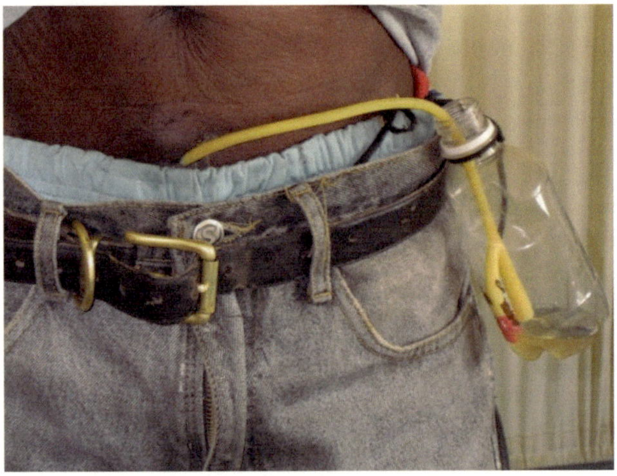

Figure 1. The patient with suprapubic catheter with abootle for drainage because there is no urine bag.

practice in settings like this. What has been noticed is that sometimes patients use to make stoppers by themselves from various materials (wood, metal, plastic) exposing themselves to the risk of infection even more.

The other factor that can promote catheter associated urinary tract infection in this setting is overinflating of the balloon of the catheter, although 10 ml of sterile water is more than enough to keep catheter in place and to make urine flow without interruption, it is not uncommon to find that the balloon is inflated with 20ml, 30ml or sometimes even more.

Overinflating the balloon may result in insufficient drainage of the bladder because of the high riding draining tip of the catheter and subsequent residual urine. The other reason to avoid overinflating of the balloon is the fact that this will inevitably lead to bladder irritation and spasms which will have an impact on the patients' quality of life.

The explanation for balloon overinflating is a rather simple one, the majority of nursing staff and junior medical staff in this setting interprets the capacity of the balloon that is indicated on the catheter as an amount of fluid that should be put in the balloon. This is also an indication of how much the urological care and education is really needed in settings like this because a great number of procedures are trained in the "see one, do one and teach one" way.

After the catheterization, we usually do not recommend antibiotics unless it is indicated for some other reason. We are trying our best in educating catheterized patient how to take care of the catheter. Regarding this matter, we teach our patients catheter care and we suggest that external genitalia should be washed on every day basis using just soap and water and at the same time the catheter itself should be washed. Teaching patients also to wash hands before any manipulation with the catheter can also minimize the risk of infection.

The other thing that we insist on is regular water intake, some 2 to $2\frac{1}{2}$ litres/day is recommended to all of our catheterized patients. These measures are rather convenient for the majority of patients and we find that the majority of patients comply with these measures.

In settings like this, one must have in mind that it is not always possible to have patients under close medical control and it is not uncommon to see catheterized patients with a catheter that has not been changed for months. Having this in mind, we find it extremely useful to insist on small, easily achievable things that can make a difference in every day urological practice.

Following these simple rules, even in settings like this, we do not see high incidence of severe infection or urosepsis due to prolonged catheterization.

When it comes to the most common pathogens isolated from our experience these are: Escherichia coli, Enterococcus spp., and Pseudomonas aeruginosa. Of course in case of long term indwelling urinary catheters, mixed bacterial pathogens are rather common.

We do not tend to treat these infections unless symptomatic, and from our experience these infections are very hard to treat due to fact that these infections are usually caused by multi-resistant bacterial pathogens. Another limiting factor is the availability of latest antibiotics.

Most common antibiotics available almost in every part of Sub-Saharan Africa are Cotrimoxazole, Nitrofurantoin and Ciprofloxacin. Thanks to the unfortunate fact that the most widely used antibiotic for almost every urological infection is Ciprofloxacin, it is not a rare case that, nowadays, bacterial resistance to this useful antibiotic is very common.

Facing all these challenges, we found that the most reliable way to prevent possible complications of CAUTI in long term catheterized patients in our setting are vigorous catheter care and proper hydration of the patient rather than unrestrained usage of precious antibiotics.

From our experience, we found that in terms of preventing CAUTI, intermittent catheterization is a much better option than long term catheterization. We found that even in our setting, it is rather easy to train patients to perform self-intermittent catheterization and to train patients for this procedure is not a demanding task. Of course, there are some limiting factors for intermittent catheterization and this is mainly because of availability of catheters, the cost of catheters and lubricating gel which are quite often out of reach for majority of patients.

The other useful thing may be proper education of nursing staff in order to become more critical when it comes to catheterization.

We should always have in mind that the patient should be catheterized only when medically indicated and never to make life easier for medical staff or family members which is, sadly, sometimes the case.

At the end, we can conclude that when it comes to catheterization and catheter associated urinary tract infection we can say that these infections, in general, are very difficult to avoid once the patient is catheterized it is only a question of time for it to occur, especially in long term catheterizations.

The things we can do to postpone CAUTI, if not avoid, in our setting would be to follow the strict indications for catheterization, to keep an indwelling catheter as short a period of time as possible and to pay attention to catheter care.

One of the major characteristics of practicing, not only Urology but Medicine in general, in Sub-Saharan Africa (Zambia) is that, due to numerous limitation factors, both medical staff and patients are forced to make the maximum out of the available resources in order to provide the best possible care.

Health care professionals should be conscious of the fact that communication should be a two-way process and that it should involve all the parties who are involved.

There is also the need for the health care professionals to educate the patients according to their individual needs.

The practical knowledge related to participants' awareness of their urinary catheter needs and practices such as features of supplies, intervals for changes, urinary catheter insertion emptying the urine bags, and changes associated with sex.

Patients living with chronic illnesses such as living with an indwelling urinary catheter are being taken care of in their homes by close relatives, whereby, they go to the hospitals only on appointments made by the doctor, for treatment and change of their catheter. Living with the indwelling urinary catheter is a condition that needs the patient to be taken care of by a skilled professional or trained personnel base in the community. Considering the lack of adequate means of communication in some parts of the country and considering the fact that not everybody can afford communicating by means of phoning, it becomes a problem to the patients in relation to the burden of illnesses and problems associated with urinary catheterization (expulsion of the urinary catheter, blockage, and leakage of urine etc.).

Health care professionals should consider their meeting with patients as a process, whereby communication should be a two-way process and not one-way; and also a time when communication should be regarded as free from imposing.

2. Education of healthcare workers

An education programme should be available at induction for new staff and on a regular basis for HCWs and should include the following:

- Indications for catheterisation.
- Insertion technique.
- Maintenance of the catheter system.
- Obtaining a urine specimen.
- Signs and symptoms of infection.
- Catheter removal

http://dx.doi.org/10.5772/55371

Author details

Mohamed Labib[1*] and Nenad Spasojevic[2]

1 Department of Surgery, School of Medicine, University of Zambia, Zambia

2 University Teaching Hospital, Lusaka, Zambia

References

[1] EAUN Evidence- based Guidelines for Best Practice in Urological Health Care 2012

[2] Emergencies in Urology : M.Hohenfellner, R.A.Santucci

[3] Catheter associated urinary tract infection is rarely symptomatic :a prospective study of 1497 catheterized patients. Arch.intern Med 160:678 : Tambyah PA, Maki DG (2000)

[4] EAU Guidelines 2012

Chapter 4

Role of Bacterial Biofilms in Catheter-Associated Urinary Tract Infections (CAUTI) and Strategies for Their Control

Mary Anne Roshni Amalaradjou and
Kumar Venkitanarayanan

Additional information is available at the end of the chapter

http://dx.doi.org/10.5772/55200

1. Introduction

Urinary tract infections (UTI's) can be defined as bacteriuria (>10^5 CFU/mL in adults; >10^4 CFU/mL in children) of an uropathogen with associated clinical signs that include dysuria and urgency [18]. According to the United States Centers for Disease Control and Prevention (CDC), a symptomatic urinary tract infection must meet at least one of the following criteria:

- Patients had/did not have an indwelling catheter in place at the time of specimen collection or onset of signs or symptoms
- Patient has at least one of the following signs or symptoms with no other recognized cause: fever (>38°C), urgency, frequency, dysuria, suprapubic tenderness or costovetebral angle pain or tenderness
- Patient has a positive urine culture of ≥10^5 with no more than 2 species of microorganisms [20].

UTI is considered to be the most common bacterial infection [107]. It is the second most common infection of any organ and is one of the most common infections in humans [157]. UTIs account for nearly 8 million physician visits and 1.5 million visits to emergency rooms annually in the United States [44, 87, 144]. Although every individual is susceptible to UTIs, certain specific subpopulations are more predisposed to the risk of UTIs. This includes infants, pregnant women, elderly, patients with spinal cord injuries and/or catheters, patients with diabetes, multiple sclerosis, or acquired immunodeficiency virus, and patients with underlying urologic abnormalities [13, 31, 43, 127, 130]. UTIs are usually localized to the bladder, kidneys or prostate. The etiology of UTIs has been regarded as well-established and consistent.

Escherichia coli is the predominant uropathogen responsible for almost 80% of all cases, followed by *Staphylococcus, Klebsiella, Enterobacter, Proteus* and *Enterococci* species [128]. The financial implications of UTIs are enormous due to high incidence. UTIs account for a total annual cost of more than $ 3.5 billion in the United States [87].

2. Catheter associated urinary tract infection

In addition to being the most common bacterial infection, UTIs are also the most common type of hospital acquired infections (HAI). HAIs can be defined as a localized or systemic condition resulting from an adverse reaction to the presence of an infectious agent or toxin, which occurs in a patient in a health care setting and was not present or incubating at the time of admission [64, 66]. UTIs account for 30% of all HAI [77]. Of these 30% infections, 80% of them are estimated to be catheter-associated [89]. According to the CDC, CAUTIs are defined as an UTI in a patient who had an indwelling urinary catheter in place at the time of or within 48 hours prior to infection onset. CAUTI can lead to complications such as cystitis, pyelonephritis, gram-negative bacteremia, prostatitis, epididymitis, endocarditis, vertebral osteomyelitis, septic arthritis, endophthalmitis and meningitis [20]. Additionally CAUTIs also result in prolonged hospital stay, increased cost and mortality [77]. An estimated 15-25% of hospitalized patients will have a urinary catheter at some point during their hospital stay [175]. Obstruction of indwelling catheters can lead to sepsis, even resulting in mortality [174]. Each year around 13,000 deaths are attributed to UTIs in the United States [77]. The cost associated with CAUTI episodes is about $750-$1000 per infection, and the estimated total cost in the United States ranges from $340-$450 million annually [132].

Millions of transurethral, suprapubic and nephrostomy catheters or urethral stents are used in patients every year. These devices overcome several host defenses and enable bacterial entry at a rate of 3 to 10% (cumulative rate) per day, which leads to bacteriuria in patients after a month [8]. In intubated patients, bacteria frequently ascend from the urethral meatus into the bladder between the mucosal and catheter surfaces. In certain cases, bacteria may ascend through the drainage system due to contamination of the drainage bag or disruption of the tubing junction. The presence of a device enables the persistence of the etiologic organism in the urinary tract. Several studies have demonstrated that bacteria exist as biofilms on these devices [53]. Formation of a biofilm and incrustation with calcium and magnesium struvites has a significant role in the pathogenesis and treatment of catheter-associated infections.

3. Biofilm

Biofilms have been around for billions of years. They have been identified in 3.2 – 3.4 billion year old South African Kornberg formation, and in deep-sea hydrothermal rocks [55]. Similar biofilms can be found in modern hot springs and deep-sea vents [124, 160]. The presence of biofilms in both ancient fossils and in similar modern environments indicates that biofilm

http://dx.doi.org/10.5772/55200

formation is an ancient and integral characteristic of prokaryotes. It is likely that biofilms provided homeostasis during the harsh and fluctuating conditions of the primitive earth such as extreme temperatures, pH and exposure to UV light, thus enabling complex interactions between individual cells. It is, however, generally accepted that planktonic cells existed before the development of biofilm communities. The concomitant development of both planktonic and sessile bacteria in biofilm communities could be attributed to the conditions offered by life on surfaces [151]. The ability of bacteria to adhere to surfaces and form biofilms in different environments is due to the selective advantage that surface association offers the bacteria.

3.1. Definition

The definition of biofilm has evolved over the years. Marshal in 1976 [94] observed the presence of fine extracellular polymer fibrils that anchored bacteria to the surface. Costerton and coworkers [1978; 28] defined biofilms as communities of attached bacteria that were found to be encased in a glycocalyx matrix of polysaccharide that mediates adhesion [28]. They also stated that biofilms consist of single cells and microcolonies which are embedded in the matrix [26]. This definition was later modified to include the ability of biofilms to adhere to surfaces and to each other forming microbial aggregates and floccules [29]. The adhesion to a surface also triggers the expression of genes controlling production of bacterial components required for biofilm formation, thus including the role of gene modulation in the definition [29]. Consequently, a definition of biofilm must include the ability of cells to attach to a surface, extrapolymeric encasing, presence of noncellular and abiotic components in the matrix, physiological attributes of these organisms and the differential gene expression in biofilm cells versus planktonic cells. Taking all this into account, biofilms can be defined as a microbially derived sessile community consisting of cells that are attached to an interface or to each other, are embedded in an extracellular polymeric matrix that they have produced and demonstrate altered phenotype associated with differential gene expression [38]. This definition also applies to biofilm cells that have broken off from a biofilm on a colonized medical device and circulate in the body fluids with the ability to establish itself in another niche.

3.2. Biofilm formation and structure

Biofilms can form on abiotic surfaces such as minerals, air-water interfaces, and biotic surfaces such as plants, other microbes and animals. In the human body, bacteria reside as biofilms on skin, oropharynx and nose, intestine and indwelling medical devices. To form a biofilm, bacteria are attracted to the surface by environmental signals. On reaching the surface, the bacteria attach to it as single cells or as clusters. When single cells attach to a surface they form a monolayer biofilm. A monolayer biofilm can be defined as one in which the bacteria attach only to the surface [75]. When bacteria attach to a surface as a cluster, they form a multilayer biofilm. Multilayer biofilms can be defined as a microbial community, where the bacteria are attached both to the surface and the neighboring bacterial cells [75]. The type of biofilm formed depends on the environmental conditions and surfaces that favor their development, the genes that are activated, the architecture of the biofilm and the matrix composition [75].

Monolayer biofilms are composed of a single layer of cells attached to a surface. These biofilms are favored when cell-surface interactions predominate. Since monolayer biofilms offer bacteria more proximity to surfaces, they commonly occur during the interaction of the bacterial pathogen with the host. In flagellate motile bacteria, monolayer formation occurs in two steps, where bacteria first become attached to a surface when they come in close proximity to it. After attachment, the bacteria break the forces tethering them to the surface, resulting in transient attachment. However, a few bacteria that have transitioned from transient to permanent attachment remain attached to the surface. Multilayer biofilms form when bacteria adhere to the surface as well as to each other. Several adhesion factors are known to mediate this transition, including preformed adhesins, conditionally synthesized adhesins and specific adhesins.

Preformed adhesins include flagellum and pili. Motility is believed to increase the initial interaction between bacteria and the surface. Several studies have also demonstrated that flagellar motility promoted surface adhesion in bacteria [76, 85, 167]. However, under certain conditions, flagellar mutants that are defective in the synthesis of flagellar components have shown an increased synthesis of adhesive matrix that promotes bacterial attachment and multilayer biofilm formation [83, 176]. These observations indicate that flagellar impedence may be important in priming the bacteria for the formation of a multilayer biofilm. Nevertheless, mutants lacking the flagellum or the flagellar motor are completely defective in monolayer and multilayer biofilm formation [83], implying that flagellar motor plays a vital role in biofilm formation independent of flagellar motility. Retractable pili are critical for gram-negative bacteria to attach to surfaces [75]. It is hypothesized that these structures pull bacteria along surfaces by attaching to the surface and retracting, thus helping the bacteria approach the surface more closely [75].

Bacteria can also conditionally synthesize adhesins to promote surface attachment. In *Pseudomonas fluorescens*, the transition from transient to permanent attachment is mediated by LapA (Large adhesion ProteinA) that associates with the bacterial surface [62]. In *E. coli*, a similar function has been attributed to the exopolysaccharide adhesin, PGA (poly-β-1,6-*N*-acetyl-d-glucosamine) which mediates the transition from temporary to permanent attachment [2]. Following the transient attachment which is accomplished through the array of adhesins such as flagella and pili, bacteria form stable and specific binding through interactions with eukaryotic cell receptors [59]. These interactions are mediated by specific adhesins which aid in internalization.

3.3. Biofilm matrix

Bacterial cells in the biofilm are surrounded by a variety of molecules that make up the matrix of the biofilm. The matrix is highly hydrated and can contain up to 97% water [154]. In addition, the matrix is composed of polysaccharides, proteins, DNA, surfactants, lipids, glycolipids, membrane vesicles and ions like calcium. This composition varies with different conditions or stages during biofilm maturation. The biofilm matrix is dynamic and interactive, and is essential to the integrity and function of the biofilm.

3.3.1. Matrix components

Exopolysaccharides are a major component of the biofilm matrix. The absence of polysaccharide synthesis and export leads to an inability to form multilayer biofilms in most bacteria. Bacteria capable of forming biofilms possess distinct genetic loci that encode for the synthesis of polysaccharides. One of the most common exopolysaccharides in the biofilm matrix is a polymer of β-1, 6-N-acteyl-D-glucosamine called PGA or PNAG. Several bacterial species, including *E. coli, S. aureus, Actinobacillus* spp., and *Bordetella* spp. make use of PGA to construct their matrix [30, 70, 71, 114, 173]. The synthesis and export of PGA is carried out by the *icaADBC* locus in Staphylococcal species and the *pgaABCS* locus in *E. coli*. PGA is required for bacterial attachment and biofilm formation in *E. coli*. Mutations in this locus prevent attachment even after prolonged incubation [173]. In *S. aureus*, the *icaADBC* locus is important for attachment and biofilm formation on indwelling medical devices [42]. In *S. epidermidis*, this locus is also shown to be required for virulence and immune evasion, thus emphasizing the role of biofilms in disease [172]. Another commonly found polysaccharide in the biofilm matrix is cellulose which has been identified as a major component of the matrix in *E. coli, Salmonella, Citrobacter, Enterobacter* and *Pseudomonas* [140, 142, 181, 182]. In *E. coli* and *Salmonella* Typhimurium, cellulose synthesis is made possible by the *bcsABZC-bcsEFG* locus [140, 182]. In addition to PGA and cellulose, some *E. coli* strains also make colanic acid, which is a branched chain polymer synthesized by the *wca* locus [146]. Mutants that are defective in colonic acid formation can attach to surfaces, but are incapable of forming multilayer biofilms [32].

The biofilm matrix is also composed of proteins exported to the matrix by cells within the biofilm. Proteinaceous appendages such as fimbriae and pili confer adhesive properties in bacteria. In *E. coli* and *Salmonella*, curli fimbriae produced by the *csgBAC* and *csgDEFG* operons are part of the biofilm matrix [57]. Transcriptional profiling studies have demonstrated that fimbria and pili gene expression is upregulated in biofilms compared to planktonic cells [12]. Another group of proteins associated with the matrix are the *Bap* or Biofilm-associated proteins. These proteins hold bacterial cells together in the biofilm by interacting with similar proteins on the surface of neighboring cells. Bap proteins have been shown to be critical for biofilm production in *S. aureus* [82]. Besides proteins that bind other proteins on neighboring cells, the biofilm matrix also contains lectins and sugar binding proteins. These proteins recognize sugar moieties on the surface of eukaryotic cells and bind to them, thereby facilitating cell-cell interactions [163]. Besides the above mentioned proteins, autotransporter proteins have been identified to be part of the biofilm matrix. The proteins can transport themselves to the cell surface without the need for other transport systems [48]. In *E. coli* autotransporters proteins such as *ag43*, AIDA and TibA have been shown to promote biofilm formation [135]. These proteins serve to maintain close-range interactions between cells in the biofilm.

Another major component of the biofilm matrix is eDNA (extracellular DNA). In *P. aeruginosa*, the biofilm matrix has significant amounts of DNA that is essential for biofilm integrity [95]. Addition of DNase to the culture media resulted in an inhibition of biofilm formation and dissolution of preformed biofilms [177]. It is hypothesized that DNA could serve as a grid that enables bacteria to move using type IV pili. The ability of type IV pili to bind DNA has been demonstrated in *P. aeruginosa* [171]. The eDNA is similar in composition to the genomic DNA, and is hypothesized to be released from whole cell lysis or secretion from outer membrane vesicles containing DNA [6].

An important characteristic of bacterial cells within the biofilm is the chemical mediated cell-cell crosstalk known as quorum sensing. Quorum sensing allows bacteria to coordinate their gene expression in a density-dependent manner [75]. These circuits involve chemical mediators or autoinducers that are secreted by the bacteria and accrue in the extracellular environment. When the autoinducer concentration exceeds a certain threshold, quorum sensing is activated. In most gram negative bacteria, the prototype quorum sensing system is the LuxI/ LuxR system [61]. LuxI proteins synthesize the autoinducer such as acylated homoserine lactone (AHL), which modulates the activity of LuxR to activate gene expression upon binding. In case of gram positive bacteria, oligopeptides serve as autoinducers which then activate gene expression in a two component system [61]. Activation of quorum sensing has been shown to stimulate biofilm formation in *P. aeruginosa*. Quorum sensing mutants of *Pseudomonas* make biofilms that are sensitive to detergents such as sodium dodecyl sulfate indicating that the matrix synthesis is defective [34]. In light of the role that quorum sensing plays in the formation and regulation of biofilms, it is proposed that use of quorum-sensing inhibitors may be a potential approach for the treatment of biofilm associated infections.

Existence as a biofilm is advantageous to the bacterium since it enables its survival under a variety of conditions. However when the environmental conditions change or their microenvironment becomes unfavorable, bacteria can return to their planktonic state. This is referred to as dispersion of biofilms. Dispersion of biofilms can be brought about by degradation of the biofilm matrix, which will lead to disruption in cell to cell adhesion and escape from the biofilm. Several bacteria have been shown to produce enzymes that can degrade matrix components and result in biofilm dispersion [15, 69]. Another mechanism of dispersion is through the induction of motility. Onset of dispersal has been shown to coincide with a return in motility of the biofilm associated cells [72]. Certain bacterial biofilms also produce surfactants such as rhamnolipids. Biofilms formed by strains of *P. aeruginosa* with increased rhamnolipid production dispersed after 2 days, whereas wild type biofilms under the same conditions did not disperse until day 10 [14]. Biofilm dispersal is of medical significance as the bacterial cells released from the biofilm can enter the body fluids and can establish themselves in another niche, thereby resulting in secondary infections.

3.4. Medical device associated biofilms

The biofilms on medical devices can be composed of gram-positive and gram-negative bacteria, or yeast. Commonly isolated bacteria include gram-positive organisms such as *E. fecalis, S. aureus, S. epidermidis, Streptococcus viridians* and gram- negative organisms like *E. coli, Klebsiella pneumonia, P. mirabilis* and *P. aeruginosa*. These organisms can reside on the skin of healthy patients or health-care workers, in the water to which entry ports are exposed or in the environment, from where they eventually contaminate the medical device. Indwelling devices can be colonized by single or multispecies biofilms. In the case of urinary catheters, initially the biofilms are composed of a single species and continued further exposures lead to multispecies biofilms [148]. There are several factors that influence the rate and extant of biofilm formation on devices. First the bacteria must attach to the surface of the device long enough to result in permanent attachment. This initial rate of attachment depends on the number and type of bacterial cells in the fluid in which the device is exposed to, the flow rate through the device and the physicochemical characteristics of the exposed surface [37]. On indwelling devices, the components in the fluid milieu to which the device is exposed to can change the surface properties and influence bacterial attachment. Following permanent attachment to the surface, the bacteria produce exopolysaccharides to form the biofilm. The rate of growth and establishment of a biofilm depends on flow rate, nutrient availability, antimicrobial concentration and temperature.

4. Urinary catheter biofilms

CAUTIs account for around 80% of all nosocomial UTIs [89]. The risk of developing an UTI significantly increases with the use of indwelling devices. It has been reported that the risk of developing CAUTI increases 5% with each day of catheterization, and virtually all patients are colonized by day 30 [91]. Several studies also support the role of biofilm in the establishment of CAUTIs [161, 167]. The predominant pathogens associated with UTIs include *E. coli* (25%), *Enterococci* (16%), *P. aeruginosa* (11%), *Klebsiella pneumonia* (8%), *Candida albicans* (8%), *Enterobacter* (5%), *P. mirabilis* (5%) and coagulase-negative *Staphylococci* (4%) [40]. These pathogens are normally found in the lower intestinal tract of humans, and can be introduced into the urinary tract via indwelling devices.

4.1. Biofilm formation on indwelling urinary tract devices

Prior to the initial attachment of bacteria to the device surface, it is critical that the surfaces are conditioned, where the attachment of proteins and polysaccharides from the fluid environment form a film on the exposed surface of the device [161, 167]. This conditioning film facilitates the initial bacterial attachment, which normally adhere poorly on uncoated surfaces [58]. Indwelling devices used in the urological settings include open and closed catheters, urethral stents and sphincters and penile prostheses. Biofilm formation has been documented from infection sites associated with all of these device types [24, 161]. Among all these devices, urinary catheters serve as the common substrate for the development of UTIs [166]. Numerous studies have demonstrated the presence of adherent biofilms on catheters removed from patients [104]. Additionally, scanning electron microscopy studies have documented extensive biofilm formation on urinary catheters [111]. Such catheters recovered from patients that failed antibiotic therapy were shown to contain *P. aeruginosa*, *E. fecalis*, *E. coli* and *P. mirabilis* [103].

4.1.1. Crystalline biofilms

Foley catheters are commonly used to manage urinary incontinence in elderly patients and those with bladder dysfunction. These devices besides helping the patient also put them under high risk for the development of UTIs. Uropathogens such as *P. mirabilis*, *Providencia stuartii*,

Morganella morganii and *K. pneumoniae* produce urease and form a unique type of crystalline biofilms on catheters. Urease production by these organisms enables them to break down the urea in urine [86] and releases ammonia, which raises the urine pH resulting in calcium and magnesium phosphate crystal formation within the biofilm matrix [149]. Studies have also demonstrated that biofilm formation is a prerequisite for crystal formation since the matrix may act as a nucleation site for crystal development [106]. Stickler and others have shown that *P. mirabilis* biofilm formation on catheter surface starts near the eye-hole in the form of microcolonies [150]. Following this, due to production of urease by these colonies, calcium and magnesium phosphate crystals begin to form and the biofilm extends down the luminal surface. The crystal formation is medically significant because of the blockage of catheters due to crystallization and encrustation, which can lead to bladder distention, urine leakage and pyelonephritis when urine from the distended bladder refluxes into the kidney. Additionally, crystalline biofilms that form on the outside of the catheter can lead to irritation and trauma of the urethral mucosa [58].

4.2. Uropathogen specific factors that contribute to biofilm formation

Uropathogenic *E. coli* (UPEC) are the most common etiology of UTIs [65]. Consequentially, UPEC biofilms are responsible for many CAUTIs [108]. Therefore this section will focus on the specific factors associated with UPEC that aid its biofilm formation. UPEC has several virulence factors such as α-hemolysin, cytotoxic necrotizing factor I, lipopolysaccharide capsule, siderphore aerobactin and enterobactin, proteases and adhesive organelles [109]. The presence of a different repertoire of virulence factors with each UPEC strain could be the reason for the high number of cases associated with UPEC [93]. The single most important virulence factor of UPEC significant to biofilm formation and the associated illness could be type I pili. Type I pili have been shown to play an important role in bacterial adhesion to biotic and abiotic surfaces, and invasion and persistence in the bladder.

Type I pili are pertrichously present on the cell surface of many members of the Enterobacteriaceae, which includes both pathogenic and commensal strains of *E. coli* [179]. Type I pili in *E. coli* is encoded by nine genes of the fim gene cluster which have structural and regulatory roles. The *fimAFGH* genes are structural genes that encode the protein components of the pilus rod and tip [58], whereas FimB and fimE encode the regulatory proteins that control phase variation of type I pili [46]. Phase variation helps *E. coli* to reversibly switch on/off the expression of type I pili, and a stringent regulation of phase variation is critical for successful UPEC infection [138]. The FimH adhesion confers mannose-specific binding property to the type I pili. FimH can recognize the terminal mannose residues on various cell types and secreted glycoproteins such as superficial bladder umbrella cells [39] and CD48 on macrophages and mast cells [136]. Langermann and others reported that FimH is essential for colonization of the murine bladder and immunization with FimH protected the animals from UPEC colonization and infection [80, 81]. Scanning electron microscopy (SEM) revealed that type I pili are in close contact with uroplakin-coated superficial bladder membrane [99]. Uroplakins are proteins that cover the apical surface of superficial umbrella cells and give strength to the bladder epithelium to create a permeability barrier [152]. *In vitro* studies using mouse uroepithelial plaques and recombinant FimH have shown that uroplakin UP1a is the unique bacterial receptor for FimH adhesion [180]. It has been shown that commensal and pathogenic *E. coli* contain type I pili and bind to trimannose receptors via FimH adhesion [139]. However, type I pili in UPEC strains also have a high affinity for binding monomannose units [180], which potentially provides a selective advantage during pathogenesis by increasing specific binding on the uroepithelium.

In addition to their role in adherence, type I pili are also essential for the invasion of bladder epithelial cells by UPEC. TEM and SEM imaging have revealed that bladder cells internalize UPEC through interactions between FimH and UP1a [99]. Other studies have also demonstrated that type I pili carrying bacteria interact with plasma membrane micro domains knows as lipid rafts [39]. More specifically, caveolae, a subtype of the lipid rafts with a cave-like appearance have been shown to associate with intracellular bacteria during UPEC invasion. Besides the bladder cells, UPEC can also bind and invade macrophages [10] and mast cells [136], thereby serving as a source of chronic UTIs. The ability of UPEC to invade macrophages allows the bacteria to survive within them and evade phagocytosis. Besides tiding over phagocytosis, ability to survive inside bladder cells also helps to avoid host defenses, including urine flow, secretion of adhesion-binding competitors such as Tamm-Horsfall protein, IgA, chemokines, and exfoliation of superficial bladder cells [113, 155]. UPEC sequestered within the bladder cells are also protected from antibiotic treatments that sterilize the urine, and are provided a rich environment in which the bacteria replicate [100]. UPEC has the ability to form biofilms on abiotic surfaces such as polypropylene, polyvinylchloride, polycarbonate and borosilicate glass when grown statically [120]. Using transposon mutagenesis, Pratt and Kolter demonstrated that Fim mutants were defective in initial attachment and biofilm formation was severely impacted. This indicates that type I pili are essential for the initial attachment of UPEC to abiotic surfaces. Besides type I pili, motility also plays an important in biofilm formation. Non motile strains were severely defective in the initial attachment and consequently in biofilm formation [120].

4.3. Biofilm formation in urinary tissues

UPEC are capable of attaching and invading uroepithelial cells, persisting and forming intracellular reservoirs that help them escape host defenses [100]. Anderson and coworkers [2003; 7] hypothesized that UPEC reservoirs are established by the formation of biofilm-like pods or intracellular bacterial communities (IBC) within the bladder cells. Replication of UPEC in the superficial bladder cells leads to the formation of tightly packed biofilm-like pods that protrude into the lumen. Bacteria inside these pods undergo continuous development leading to the maturation of the IBCs. The development of IBC can be divided into four phases. The first phase begins 1-3 h after infection. The type I pili bind and invade the superficial bladder epithelial cells [74]. At this stage the bacteria are non-motile and divide rapidly and by 8 h post infection, they form loosely organized colonies that resemble microcolonies of abiotic biofilms, known as early IBC. The next phase leads to the formation of middle IBCs, which is characterized by a reduction in cell proliferation and cell size. Each pod corresponds to a single epithelial cell tightly packed with bacteria forming an intracellular biofilm. Within the pods, a polysaccharide matrix surrounds the bacteria [7, 74]. At around 12 h post infection, late IBCs are formed, when UPEC regain their rod shape and motility and flux out of the bladder cells. Fluxing aids UPEC in infecting neighboring cells [74]. The last phase of IBC formation results in UPEC filamentation which occurs 24 to 48 h post infection, where filamentation helps UPEC evade host immune responses. The filamentous bacteria can also separate to form rod-shaped daughter cells. The appearance of filamentous cells also coincides with the appearance of small groups of UPEC on newly infected healthy cells [74].

4.3.1. Pathogenesis of catheter-associated biofilm

The pathogenesis of CAUTI depends on the physicochemical properties of the catheter material and its susceptibility to bacterial colonization. Bacterial binding to the bladder mucosa triggers an inflammatory response that leads to neutrophil influx and sloughing of the infected epithelial cells [78]. This helps to clear the bacteria from the mucosal surface. In the case of a catheter, besides the absence of inherent defense mechanisms, they also provide a survival advantage to the bacteria which become difficult to eradicate. The advantages include resistance from being swept away by the urine flow, resistance to phagocytosis and antimicrobials [167]. In addition to the catheter providing an environment for biofilm formation, the presence of a catheter helps to weaken many normal defenses of the bladder. The catheter helps to connect the heavily colonized perineum with the sterile bladder, thus providing a route for bacterial entry into the bladder. Urine pools in the bladder or in the catheter and the resulting urinary stasis promote bacterial growth. Additionally, the catheter also damages the bladder mucosa by triggering inflammatory response and mechanical erosion [175]. Once bacteria gain entry into the urinary tract, low level bacteriuria progresses within 24 to 48 h in the absence of an antimicrobial therapy [145].

4.4. Biofilm related UTIs

Chronic bacterial prostatitis: The prostatic ducts and acini provide a safe environment for bacteria to multiply and induce host response. If the bacteria are not eradicated by the immune response, it leads to their persistence and formation of bacterial microcolonies. The presence of microcolonies induces persistent immunological stimulation and chronic inflammation [105].

Recurrent cystitis: UPEC binds to superficial bladder epithelial cells resulting in neutrophil recruitment and influx into the bladder lumen. Neutrophil recruitment occurs due to the recognition of bacterial LPS by the toll-like receptors. Additionally, interaction between type I pili and the uroepithelium results in exfoliation of the superficial epithelial cells causing pathogen shedding into the urine [129]. When IBCs form in the epithelial cells, they persist as a chronic reservoir, which leads to recurrent cystitis.

Pyelonephritis: Once the bacteria reach the kidney, they adhere to the uroepithelium and form thin biofilms before invading the renal tissue [106]. Additionally encrustation and obstruction to the catheter flow due to formation of crystalline biofilms leads to bladder distention, urine leakage and pyelonephritis when urine from the distended bladder refluxes in to the kidney [162].

Infected urinary caliculi: In case of urease positive bacteria, biofilm formation is accompanied by the deposition of calcium and magnesium crystals. This crystallization occurs only after the biofilm is formed, since the biofilm serves as a nucleation site [106].

5. Control strategies to prevent CAUTI

CAUTI is the most common hospital acquired infection and accounts for up to 40% of all health care associated infections in the United States [102, 156]. About 15-25% of hospitalized patients have an urethral catheter in place during some point of their stay. It is estimated that around 30 million bladder catheters are placed annually in the United States, resulting in several hundred thousand cases of CAUTI [156]. A systemic review of the proportion of health care associated infections that can be prevented revealed that CAUTI was the most preventable nosocomial infection [170]. An estimate of the number of avoidable cases ranged from 95,483 to 387,550 per year and associated lives saved ranged from 2225 to 9031 annually. This prevention could also avoid the annual cost of these illnesses which is estimated at $1.8 million to $115 million [170]. This underscores the need for control strategies to prevent CAUTI. Prevention of CAUTI is primarily based on reviewing the criteria for appropriate placement and early removal of catheters. The advances in our understanding of the pathogenesis and key factors that influence the onset of infection are also critical in the development of adequate and effective control strategies [137]. Several protective strategies have been suggested for CAUTI, some of which are already in place for patient care, whereas others are still in development. The control strategies include:

5.1. Need for and duration of catheterization

It is estimated that about 21-50% of catheters are placed without justified need and catheters are inappropriately retained for 33-50% of total device days [73, 101]. The most effective ways for the preventing CAUTI are by reducing the duration of catheterization and its early removal [51]. Use of interventions such as nurse prompted removal suggestions and computer based reminders to the patients have resulted in a decline in catheter retention and a concomitant reduction in bacteriuria [164]. Thus, it is important to refrain from using an indwelling catheter without an appropriate indication. A study conducted in an emergency department indicated that use of pre-insertion checklists have led to an improved adherence to indications for placement resulting in the increase in the number of appropriately placed catheters from 37% to 51% [50].

5.2. Catheter placement and management

Since the catheter provides a connection between the highly colonized perineum and the sterile bladder, sterility during catheter handling and placement is of greatest importance. In this regard, hand hygiene plays a vital role in the prevention of CAUTI [16]. Insertion of a catheter in the emergency room rather than an operating room has been shown to be associated with higher rates of catheter associated bacteriuria (CAB; 158). Use of an aseptic insertion technique reduces the risk of acquiring resistant organisms in the hospital [63]. A randomized study conducted by Platt and others [1983; 118] demonstrated that hospitalized patients intubated with a catheter without a pre-sealed junction were 2.7 times more likely to develop CAB than patients with pre-connected catheter drainage bags and sealed junctions. Therefore, the use of closed catheter drainage systems universally is recommended [63]. Similarly, any breach in the closed drainage system would also increase the risk for CAB. Any manipulation of the indwelling catheter should be avoided so that breaches in the closed drainage and shear trauma can be minimized [25].

5.3. Catheter design

Catheter design has not changed significantly since the inception of the Foley catheter in the 1930s [97]. In addition to the catheter design, biocompatibility of the material is crucial. Catheter material can also impact the rate of biofilm formation. Scanning electron microscopy imaging of latex catheters revealed that presence of more uneven surfaces on it than other silicone counterparts which can promote bacterial adhesion [150]. Additionally latex has been associated with toxic effects *in vitro* and proinflammatory reactions *in vivo* leading to polypoid cystitis on chronic exposure [49]. Moreover, silicone catheters are more popular to avoid allergic reactions associated with latex use. Besides being hypoallergenic, silicone catheters have a larger lumen and are minimally prone to encrustation by crystalline biofilms [36]. A newly engineered silicone catheter with a trefoil cross-section was shown to reduce CAB and inflammation when compared to a standard urinary catheter [153]. The trefoil conformation helps to minimize the surface area of contact between the catheter and the urethra, thereby decreasing friction and trauma and increasing drainage of urethral secretions [137].

5.4. Hydrogel coated catheters

Cross linked insoluble polymers that are hydrophilic and trap water are known as hydrogels. Use of hydrophilic coating on catheters has been shown to improve patient comfort, reduce bacterial adherence and encrustation. The presence of hydrogels also increases lubrication and decreases bacterial adhesion to the interface of the tissue and the catheter [11]. However, conflicting data exist on the ability of hydrogel coated catheters to reduce CAUTI, which could be attributed to the type of hydrogel incorporated. Tunney and Gorman [2002; 169] used *in vitro* models to demonstrate that Poly(vinyl pyrollidone)-coated polyurethane catheters had a lower rate of encrustation when compared to uncoated polyurethane and silicone catheters. Another study showed that the use of poly(ethylene oxide)-based multiblock copolymer and segmented polyurethane increased the time to encrustation and catheter blockage from 7.8 h to 20.1 h [116]. These findings collectively suggest that the type of hydrogel coating can affect the rate of encrustation and the resulting catheter blockage.

http://dx.doi.org/10.5772/55200

5.5. Antimicrobial coating

Antimicrobial modification of catheters is achieved by coating, matrix loading and immersion in an antimicrobial solution. The primary objective behind the incorporation of antimicrobial on a catheter is to reduce bacterial attachment and biofilm formation. Additionally, release of antimicrobials from the catheters into the milieu is also another potential approach to control planktonic cells of uropathogens [56].

5.5.1. *Nanoparticles and iontophoresis*

Nanoparticles by virtue of their small size have the ability to penetrate bacterial cells, disrupt cell membranes and bind to the chromosomal DNA. Lelouche and others [2009; 84] demonstrated that glass surfaces coated with magnesium fluoride nanoparticles inhibited biofilm formation by *S. aureus* and *E. coli*, whereas magnesium fluoride solutions did not affect biofilm formation. This highlights the size dependent effect of nanoparticles.

The application of low intensity direct current (Ionotophoresis) *in vitro* has been shown to increase the antimicrobial activity of antibiotics on bacteria embedded in biofilms [27]. Chakravarti and others [2005; 21] used a urinary flow model to test the *in vitro* antibiofilm efficacy of iontophoretic silver wire containing silicone catheters. These catheters were challenged with *P. mirabilis* and then exposed to a steady current of 150 μA. It was observed that application of the electric field increased the time to blockage from 22 h to 156 h, and reduced the viable count from 10^9 CFU/ml to 10^4 CFU/ml. Similar *in vivo* study in sheep intubated with catheters containing platinum electrodes showed a decline in pathogen count from 10^7 CFU/ml to 10^3 CFU/ml on application of a direct current of 400 μA [33].

5.5.2. *Antimicrobials*

A variety of antimicrobials applied on urinary catheters have been investigated for their efficacy in controlling UTIs using *in vitro* and *in vivo* models.Nitrous oxide is known to exhibit bactericidal activity [123]. Urinary catheters impregnated with gaseous nitrous oxide, a known antimicrobial, and challenged with *E. coli* resulted in the slow release of nitrous oxide into the urine for over 14 days, and decreased biofilm formation by *E. coli*. Chlorhexidine is a common antimicrobial used against oral plaques. *In vivo* studies in rabbits intubated with genidine (combination of chlorhexidine and gentian violet) coated silicone catheters showed a reduction in biofilm formation by *E. coli, E. faecium, P. aeruginosa, K. pneumoniae* and *Candida* in comparison to silver coated and uncoated catheters [54]. Catheter associated bacteriuria was noticed in 60% and 71% of the rabbits with uncoated catheters and silver hydrogel coated catheters, respectively, whereas CAB did not occur in any of the rabbits with genidine coated catheters. Similar to chlorhexidine, triclosan is another antibacterial ingredient in toothpastes and cleaners used in health care settings. Triclosan exerts its antibacterial effect by inhibiting bacterial fatty acid synthesis [147]. Incorporation of triclosan in the balloon of catheters resulted in its release and diffusion through latex and silicon catheter balloons. The balloon served as a reservoir and the membrane helped in controlled release of triclosan. This in turn slowed encrustation and maintained the lumen patent for 7 days as compared to 24 h in saline-filled catheters [150]. Another antibacterial shown to possess antibiofilm effect is nitrofurazone, which interferes with bacterial ribosomes, DNA and cell wall. When nitrofurazone coated catheters were compared with standard catheters, it was observed that nitrofurazone significantly reduced CAB [133]. Besides nitrofurazone, norfloxacin coated catheters were also shown to inhibit the growth of *E. coli, K. pneumoniae* and *P. vulgaris* for up to 10 days [115]. Similarly, gentamicin coated catheters were also effective in reducing CAB in rabbits [23]. Another study demonstrated that sparfloxacin coated and heparin coated catheters reduced colonization by *S. aureus, E. coli* and *S. epidermidis* for greater than 26 days compared to control catheters [79]. However, the use of antibiotics on catheters to control bacterial biofilms could potentially lead to the emergence of antibiotic resistant bacteria [126]. Repeated use of antibiotics for treating UTIs has been linked to the emergence of antibiotic resistant UPEC [41, 126]. Therefore, there is an increasing interest in the use of natural antimicrobials for controlling microbial infections, including UTIs.

5.5.3. Plant molecules

Plants are capable of synthesizing a large number of molecules [47], most of which are produced as a defense mechanism against predation by microorganisms and insects. A variety of plant-derived polyphenols are active components in traditional medicines [178]. A significant body of literature exists on the positive effects of dietary intake of berry fruits on human health, performance and disease [134]. Cranberry products such as its juice and tablets have been used as an alternative medicine to prevent UTIs in humans for decades. Clinical and epidemiological studies support the use of cranberry in maintaining a healthy urinary tract [117]. Although several studies have tested the antimicrobial effect of cranberries against multiple uropathogens, it was found to be most effective against UPEC.

Cranberries exert anti-adhesive effects on certain uropathogens [112] and this effect is specific to certain components of cranberry [110]. Cranberries contain three different flavonoids (flavonols, anthocyanins and PAC), catechins, hydroxycinnamic and other phenolic acids and triterpenoids. The anthocyanins are absorbed in the human circulatory system and transported without any chemical change to the urine [117]. Cranberry products do not inhibit bacterial growth, but reduced bacterial adherence to uroepithelial cells, thereby decreasing the development of UTI. The anti-adhesive effects of p-fimbriated UPEC to uroepithelial cells are related with A-linked PAC as compared with lack of anti-adhesion activities of B-linked PAC from grape, apple juice, green tea and chocolate [67]. The A-type PAC in cranberries enhances the anti-adhesive effects *in vitro* and in urine. PAC binds to lipopolysaccharide in gram-negative bacteria. When *E. coli* was grown in the presence of cranberry components, the bacterial morphology changed to a more spherical cell-like form. These changes cause them to be repelled by the human cells [88]. Similar study by Tao and others [2011; 159] have also demonstrated that consumption of cranberry juice cocktail reduced the adhesion of UPEC to a silicon nitride probe.

Cranberry has undergone extensive evaluation in the management of UTIs. However, currently there is no evidence that cranberry can be used to treat UTIs. Hence, the focus has been on its use as a prophylactic agent in the prevention of UTIs [52]. The consumption of cranberry juice can help to prevent the adhesion of UPEC to the uroepithelium and thereby help reduce the incidence of UTIs. With rising concerns of antibiotic resistance among UPEC, cranberry could serve as an effective alternative in controlling UTIs.

Trans-cinnamaldehyde (TC) is a major component of the bark extract of cinnamon [1]. It is a generally recognized as safe (GRAS) molecule approved for use in foods by the Food and Drug Administration (FDA). The U. S. Flavoring Extract Manufacturers' Association reported that TC has a wide margin of safety between conservative estimates of intake and no observed adverse effect levels, from sub-chronic and chronic studies [1]. The report also indicated no genotoxic or mutagenic effects due to TC. Although, cinnamon or cinnamon oil has been used for ages in the treatment of UTIs, no scientific study was undertaken to investigate its antimicrobial efficacy against uropathogens. Amalaradjou and group [2010; 4] investigated the efficacy of TC for controlling UPEC biofilm formation. They observed that TC as a catheter lock solution or as a coating significantly inactivated UPEC and prevented biofilm formation when compared to untreated catheters. In a follow up study, these researchers reported that TC decreased the attachment and invasion of UPEC in cultured urinary tract epithelial cells by down-regulating several virulence genes in the pathogen [5].

Besides the use of cranberry and TC, other plant derived natural antimicrobials have also been shown to be effective against uropathogens. Sosa and Zunino [2009; 141] demonstrated that *Ibicella lutea* (Devils claw or Rams horn) extracts had an effect on bacterial growth rate and morphology of *P.mirabilis* by affecting its swarming differentiation, hemagglutination and biofilm formation on glass and polystyrene. Similarly, the use of *Coccinia grandis* (Ivy gourd) plant extracts have been reported to inhibit growth of UPEC *in vitro* [119]. Several other herbs that are used for the treatment of UTIs, but lacking scientific basis include *Agrimonia eupatoria* (agrimony), *Althea officinalis* (marshmallow), *Apium graveolens* (celery seed), *Arctium lappa* (burdock), *Elymus repens* (couchgrass), *Hydrangea aborescens* (hydrangea), *Juniperus communis* (juniper), *Mentha piperita* (peppermint), *Taraxacum officinalis* leaf (dandelion), *Ulmus fulva* (slippery elm) and *Zea mays* (corn silk; 3).

5.5.4. Silver coated catheters

Silver is a well-known antimicrobial exerting its bactericidal action by inactivating bacterial enzymes and causing cell wall damage [96]. Silver alloy and silver oxide coatings on catheters were investigated for reducing CAB, where silver alloy coating was found to be more effective [131]. In addition to reducing CAB, other studies also demonstrated the ability of silver alloy to decrease CAUTI compared to silver oxide or latex catheters [143]. However other researchers have observed conflicting results with no difference in antibiofilm effect of silver alloy and silver oxide [122, 143].

5.6. Enzyme inhibitors

Urease producing bacteria are known to produce crystalline biofilms and encrustation on catheters. Use of urease inhibitors such as acetohydroxamic acid and fluorofamide have been reported to reduce encrustation and thereby prevent CAB [98]. These urease inhibitors have been also shown to prevent urea break down and pH increase *in vitro* by *P. mirabilis* besides decreasing the associated encrustation. Another enzyme target is N-acetyl-D-glucosamine-1-phosphate acetyltransferase, which is essential for peptidoglycan, lipopolysaccharide and adhesion synthesis. Inhibitors of the enzyme belonging to the N-substituted maleimide family have produced antibiofilm activity against *P. aeruginosa* and *S. epidermidis* compared to silver hydrogel coated catheters [17].

5.6.1. Bacterial interference

Use of nonpathogenic microorganisms to counteract pathogenic bacteria is known as bacterial interference [137]. Colonization of catheter surfaces with nonpathogenic bacteria can prevent adhesion and colonization by pathogens. The nonpathogenic *E. coli* 83972 has been extensively investigated both *in vitro* and *in vivo* in bacterial interference protocols [68]. Initially, studies with this nonpathogenic strain were done by instilling the bacteria into the bladder of patients. Colonization by *E. coli* 83972 protected these patients from symptomatic UTI. To reduce the need for instillation of bacteria into the bladder of patients, experiments were later conducted with catheters coated with the nonpathogenic strain [168]. This study also revealed that *E. coli* 83972 was effective in reducing symptomatic UTI similar to previous experiments with direct infusion of the bacteria.

5.6.2. Bacteriophages

Another potential approach investigated for controlling CAUTI is the use of bacteriophages. Catheters coated with T4 bacteriophage against *E. coli* and coli-proteus bacteriophage active against Proteus were exposed to *E. coli* ATCC 11303, *P. mirabilis* or saline. It was observed that phage treatment of catheters led to approximately 90% reduction in biofilm formation compared to control catheters [19]. It was also observed that the application of phage cocktail on catheters was more effective against bacteria than the use of a single phage [19]. When hydrogel coated catheters were pretreated with a five-phage cocktail, *P. aeruginosa* biofilm formation was reduced by 99% after 48 h [45].

5.6.3. Liposomes

Liposomes are carrier or delivery vehicles that can carry both hydrophilic and hydrophobic molecules to their target site for delivery. This helps to increase the half life of the drugs besides protecting them from the environment. Liposomes containing ciprofloxacin embedded in a hydrogel coated catheter were evaluated in a rabbit model to investigate its antibiofilm effect against *E. coli* induced CAUTI [121]. The results from this study revealed that liposomal ciprofloxacin treated group had a delayed onset of positive urine cultures compared to the control group.

5.6.4. Quorum sensing inhibitors

Quorum sensing between bacterial cells in a biofilm have been shown to be essential for biofilm formation and maintenance. Inhibition of quorum sensing could therefore provide a potential route for the control of biofilms. *Delisea pulchra,* an algal species has been shown to produce furanones that interfere with autoinducer signaling and biofilm formation [92]. *In vitro* and *in vivo* sheep experiments using furanone containing catheters have been evaluated against *S. epidermidis* [35]. Similarly, use of azithromycin has been shown to inhibit the production of quorum sensing signals, swimming, swarming and twitching motilities, and biofilm formation *in vitro* [9].

5.6.5. Surface vibroacoustic stimulation

Catheters containing peizo elements can generate low energy acoustic waves that can lead to the formation of a vibrating coat along the catheter and prevent bacterial attachment and biofilm formation [60]. Scanning electron microscopy studies demonstrated that application of surface acoustic waves led to reduced biofilm formation by *E. coli, E. faecalis, Candida albicans* and *P. mirabilis*. An *in vivo* study in rabbits demonstrated that peizo element containing catheters with acoustic vibration led to a delayed positive urine culture compared to control animals [60]. The acoustic waves generated resulted in bacterial vibration at the same frequency, thereby preventing bacterial attachment and eventual biofilm formation.

6. Conclusion

Catheter associated urinary tract infections are the most common nosocomial infections and a vast majority of them are caused by biofilms formed on catheters. The complications caused by biofilms can undermine the patient's quality of life and threaten their health. The high incidence of CAUTI and the consequent complications warrants the development and application of effective control strategies. Prevention is predominantly based on enforcing guidelines for appropriate catheter placement and early removal. However, a comprehensive understanding of bacterial biofilm formation, pathogenesis and other key factors essential for development of UTIs would help in the development of novel and effective control strategies.

Author details

Mary Anne Roshni Amalaradjou[1] and Kumar Venkitanarayanan[2]

*Address all correspondence to: kumar.venkitanarayanan@uconn.edu

1 Department of Food Science, Purdue University, West Lafayette, IN, USA

2 Department of Animal Science, University of Connecticut, Storrs, CT, USA

References

[1] Adams TB, Cohen SM, Doull J, Feron VJ, Goodman JI, Marnett LJ, Munro IC, Portoghese PS, Smith RL, Waddell WJ, Wagner BM. The FEMA GRAS assessment of cinnamyl derivatives used as flavor ingredients. Food Chem Toxicol 2004: 42:157-185.

[2] Agladze K, Wang X, Romeo T. Spatial periodicity of *Escherichia coli* K-12 biofilm microstructure initiates during a reversible, polar attachment phase of development and requires the polysaccharide adhesin PGA. J Bacteriol 2005;187:8237-46.

[3] Amalaradjou MAR, Venkitanarayanan K. (2011). Natural Approaches for Controlling Urinary Tract Infections, Urinary Tract Infections, Peter Tenke (Ed.), ISBN: 978-953-307-757-4, InTech, Available from: http://www.intechopen.com/books/urinary-tract-infections/natural-approaches-for-controlling-urinary-tract-infections

[4] Amalaradjou MA, Narayanan A, Baskaran SA, Venkitanarayanan K. Antibiofilm effect of trans-cinnamaldehyde on uropathogenic *Escherichia coli*. J Urol, 2010: 184:358-363.

[5] Amalaradjou MA, Narayanan A, Venkitanarayanan K. Trans-cinnamaldehyde decreases attachment and invasion of uropathogenic *Escherichia coli* in urinary tract epithelial cells by modulating virulence gene expression. J Urol 2011;185:1526-1531.

[6] Allesen-Holm M, Barken KB, Yang L, Klausen M, Webb JS, Kjelleberg S, et al. A characterization of DNA release in Pseudomonas aeruginosa cultures and biofilms. Mol Microbiol 2006;59:1114-28.

[7] Anderson GG, Palermo JJ, Schilling JD, Roth R, Heuser J, Hultgren SJ. Intracellular bacterial biofilm-like pods in urinary tract infections. Science 2003;301:105-7.

[8] Bagshaw SM, Laupland KB. Epidemiology of intensive care unit-acquired urinary tract infections. Curr Opin Infect Dis 2006;19:67-71.

[9] Bala A, Kumar R, Harjai K. Inhibition of quorum sensing in *Pseudomonas aeruginosa* by azithromycin and its effectiveness in urinary tract infections. J Med Microbiol. 2011;60:300-6.

[10] Baorto DM, Gao Z, Malaviya R, Dustin ML, van der Merwe A, Lublin DM, et al. Survival of FimH-expressing enterobacteria in macrophages relies on glycolipid traffic. Nature 1997;389:636-9.

[11] Beiko DT, Knudsen BE, Watterson JD, Cadieux PA, Reid G, Denstedt JD. Urinary tract biomaterials. J Urol 2004;171:2438-44.

[12] Beloin C, Valle J, Latour-Lambert P, Faure P, Kzreminski M, Balestrino D, et al. Global impact of mature biofilm lifestyle on Escherichia coli K-12 gene expression. Mol Microbiol 2004;51:659-74.

[13] Biering-Sørensen F, Bagi P, Høiby N. Urinary tract infections in patients with spinal cord lesions: treatment and prevention. Drugs 2001;61:1275-87.

[14] Boles BR, Thoendel M, Singh PK. Rhamnolipids mediate detachment of Pseudomonas aeruginosa from biofilms. Mol Microbiol 2005;57:1210-23.

[15] Boles BR, Horswill AR. Agr-mediated dispersal of *Staphylococcus aureus* biofilms. PLoS Pathog 2008;4(4):e1000052.

[16] Boyce JM, Pittet D. Guideline for Hand Hygiene in Health-Care Settings. Recommendations of the Healthcare Infection Control Practices Advisory Committee and the HICPAC/SHEA/APIC/IDSA Hand Hygiene Task Force. Society for Healthcare Epidemiology of America/Association for Professionals in Infection Control/Infectious Diseases Society of America.; Healthcare Infection Control Practices Advisory Committee; HICPAC/SHEA/APIC/IDSA Hand Hygiene Task Force. MMWR Recomm Rep 2002;51(RR-16):1-45.

[17] Burton E, Gawande PV, Yakandawala N, LoVetri K, Zhanel GG, Romeo T, et al. Antibiofilm activity of GlmU enzyme inhibitors against catheter-associated uropathogens. Antimicrob Agents Chemother 2006;50:1835-40.

[18] Burckhardt I, Zimmermann S. *Streptococcus pneumoniae* in urinary tracts of children with chronic kidney disease. Emerg Infect Dis 2011;17(1):120-2.

[19] Carson L, Gorman SP, Gilmore BF. The use of lytic bacteriophages in the prevention and eradication of biofilms of *Proteus mirabilis* and Escherichia coli. FEMS Immunol Med Microbiol 2010;59:447-55.

[20] Centers for Disease Control. 2012. Device- associated module: Catheter associated urinary tract infection event. http://www.cdc.gov/nhsn/pdfs/pscmanual/7psccauti-current.pdf

[21] Chakravarti A, Gangodawila S, Long MJ, Morris NS, Blacklock AR, Stickler DJ. An electrified catheter to resist encrustation by *Proteus mirabilis* biofilm. J Urol 2005;174:1129-32.

[22] Chenworth CE, Saint S. Urinary tract infections. Infect Dis Clin North Am 2011; 25(1):103-115.

[23] Cho YW, Park JH, Kim SH, Cho YH, Choi JM, Shin HJ, et al. Gentamicin-releasing urethral catheter for short-term catheterization. J Biomater Sci Polym Ed 2003;14:963-72.

[24] Choong S, Whitfield H. Biofilms and their role in infections in urology. BJU Int 2000;86:935-41.

[25] Classen DC, Larsen RA, Burke JP, Stevens LE. Prevention of catheter-associated bacteriuria: clinical trial of methods to block three known pathways of infection. Am J Infect Control 1991;19(3):136-42.

[26] Costerton JW, Cheng KJ, Geesey GG, Ladd TI, Nickel JC, Dasgupta M, et al. Bacterial biofilms in nature and disease. Annu Rev Microbiol 1987;41:435-64.

[27] Costerton JW, Ellis B, Lam K, Johnson F, Khoury AE. Mechanism of electrical enhancement of efficacy of antibiotics in killing biofilm bacteria. Antimicrob Agents Chemother 1994;38:2803-9.

[28] Costerton JW, Geesey GG, Cheng KJ. How bacteria stick. Sci Am 1978;238:86-95.

[29] Costerton JW, Lewandowski Z, Caldwell DE, Korber DR, Lappin-Scott HM. Microbial biofilms. Annu Rev Microbiol 1995;49:711-45.

[30] Cramton SE, Gerke C, Schnell NF, Nichols WW, Götz F. The intercellular adhesion (ica) locus is present in *Staphylococcus aureus* and is required for biofilm formation. Infect Immun 1999;67:5427-33.

[31] Cunningham FG, Lucas MJ. Urinary tract infections complicating pregnancy. Baillieres Clin Obstet Gynaecol 1994;8:353-73.

[32] Danese PN, Pratt LA, Kolter R. Exopolysaccharide production is required for development of Escherichia coli K-12 biofilm architecture. J Bacteriol 2000;182:3593-6.

[33] Davis CP, Shirtliff ME, Scimeca JM, Hoskins SL, Warren MM. In vivo reduction of bacterial populations in the urinary tract of catheterized sheep by iontophoresis. J Urol 1995;154:1948-53.

[34] Davies DG, Parsek MR, Pearson JP, Iglewski BH, Costerton JW, Greenberg EP. The involvement of cell-to-cell signals in the development of a bacterial biofilm. Science. 1998;280(5361):295-8.

[35] de Nys R, Givskov M, Kumar N, Kjelleberg S, Steinberg PD. Furanones. Prog Mol Subcell Biol 2006;42:55-86.

[36] Denstedt JD, Wollin TA, Reid G. Biomaterials used in urology: current issues of biocompatibility, infection, and encrustation. J Endourol 1998;12:493-500.

[37] Donlan RM. Biofilms and device-associated infections. Emerg Infect Dis 2001;7:277-81.

[38] Donlan RM, Costerton JW. Biofilms: survival mechanisms of clinically relevant microorganisms. Clin Microbiol Rev 2002;15:167-93.

[39] Duncan MJ, Li G, Shin JS, Carson JL, Abraham SN. Bacterial penetration of bladder epithelium through lipid rafts. J Biol Chem 2004;279:18944-51.

[40] Emori TG, Gaynes RP. An overview of nosocomial infections, including the role of the microbiology laboratory. Clin Microbiol Rev 1993;6(4):428-42.

[41] Farshad S, Japoni A, Hosseini M. Low distribution of integrons among multidrug resistant E. coli strains isolated from children with community-acquired urinary tract infections in Shiraz, Iran. Pol J Microbiol 2008;57(3):193-8.

[42] Fluckiger U, Ulrich M, Steinhuber A, Döring G, Mack D, Landmann R, et al. Biofilm formation, icaADBC transcription, and polysaccharide intercellular adhesin synthesis by staphylococci in a device-related infection model. Infect Immun 2005;73:1811-9.

[43] Foxman B. Epidemiology of urinary tract infections: incidence, morbidity, and economic costs. Am J Med 2002;113 Suppl 1A:5S-13S.

[44] Foxman B. Epidemiology of urinary tract infections: incidence, morbidity, and economic costs. Dis. Mon 2003; 49: 53-70.

[45] Fu W, Forster T, Mayer O, Curtin JJ, Lehman SM, Donlan RM. Bacteriophage cocktail for the prevention of biofilm formation by Pseudomonas aeruginosa on catheters in an in vitro model system. Antimicrob Agents Chemother 2010;54:397-404.

[46] Gally DL, Leathart J, Blomfield IC. Interaction of FimB and FimE with the fim switch that controls the phase variation of type 1 fimbriae in Escherichia coli K-12. Mol Microbiol 1996;21:725-38.

[47] Geissman TA. *(*1963*)* Flavonoid compounds, tannins, lignins and related compounds. *in Pyrrole pigments, isoprenoid compounds and phenolic plant constituents, eds* Florkin M., Stotz E. H. *(*Elsevier, New York, N.Y*)*, 9*:*265.

[48] Girard V, Mourez M. Adhesion mediated by autotransporters of Gram-negative bacteria: structural and functional features. Res Microbiol 2006;157:407-16.

[49] Goble NM, Clarke T, Hammonds JC. Histological changes in the urinary bladder secondary to urethral catheterisation. Br J Urol 1989;63:354-7.

[50] Gokula RM, Smith MA, Hickner J. Emergency room staff education and use of a urinary catheter indication sheet improves appropriate use of Foley catheters. Am J Infect Control 2007;35:589-93.

[51] Griffiths R, Fernandez R. Strategies for the removal of short-term indwelling urethral catheters in adults. Cochrane Database Syst Rev 2007:CD004011.

[52] Guay DRP. Cranberry and urinary tract infections. Drugs 2009;69: 775-807.

[53] Guggenbichler JP, Assadian O, Boeswald M, Kramer A. Incidence and clinical implication of nosocomial infections associated with implantable biomaterials - catheters, ventilator-associated pneumonia, urinary tract infections. GMS Krankenhhyg Interdiszip 2011;6:Doc18.

[54] Hachem R, Reitzel R, Borne A, Jiang Y, Tinkey P, Uthamanthil R, et al. Novel antiseptic urinary catheters for prevention of urinary tract infections: correlation of in vivo and in vitro test results. Antimicrob Agents Chemother 2009;53:5145-9.

[55] Hall-Stoodley L, Costerton JW, Stoodley P. Bacterial biofilms: from the natural environment to infectious diseases. Nat Rev Microbiol 2004;2:95-108.

[56] Hamill TM, Gilmore BF, Jones DS, Gorman SP. Strategies for the development of the urinary catheter. Expert Rev Med Devices 2007;4:215-25.

[57] Hammar M, Arnqvist A, Bian Z, Olsén A, Normark S. Expression of two csg operons is required for production of fibronectin- and congo red-binding curli polymers in Escherichia coli K-12. Mol Microbiol 1995;18:661-70.

[58] Hatt JK, Rather PN. Role of bacterial biofilms in urinary tract infections. Curr Top Microbiol Immunol 2008;322:163-92.

[59] Hauck CR. Cell adhesion receptors - signaling capacity and exploitation by bacterial pathogens. Med Microbiol Immunol 2002;191:55-62.

[60] Hazan Z, Zumeris J, Jacob H, Raskin H, Kratysh G, Vishnia M, et al. Effective prevention of microbial biofilm formation on medical devices by low-energy surface acoustic waves. Antimicrob Agents Chemother 2006;50:4144-52.

[61] Henke JM, Bassler BL. Bacterial social engagements. Trends Cell Biol 2004;14:648-56.

[62] Hinsa SM, Espinosa-Urgel M, Ramos JL, O'Toole GA. Transition from reversible to irreversible attachment during biofilm formation by Pseudomonas fluorescens WCS365 requires an ABC transporter and a large secreted protein. Mol Microbiol 2003;49:905-18.

[63] Hooton TM, Bradley SF, Cardenas DD, Colgan R, Geerlings SE, Rice JC, et al. Diagnosis, prevention, and treatment of catheter-associated urinary tract infection in adults: 2009 International Clinical Practice Guidelines from the Infectious Diseases Society of America. Clin Infect Dis 2010;50:625-63.

[64] Hooton TM, Carlet JM, Duse AG, Krieger JN, Steele L, Sunakawa K. (2001) Definitions and epidemiology. In: Naber KG, Pechere JC, Kumazawa J, Khoury S, Gerberding JL, Schaeffer AJ (eds) Nosocomial and Health Care Associated Infections in Urology. Health Publication, Plymouth

[65] Hooton TM, Stamm WE. Diagnosis and treatment of uncomplicated urinary tract infection. Infect Dis Clin North Am 1997;11:551-81.

[66] Horan TC, Andrus M, Dudeck MA. CDC/NHSN surveillance definition of health care-associated infection and criteria for specific types of infections in the acute care setting. Am J Infect Control 2008;36:309-32.

[67] Howell AB, Reed JD, Krueger CG, Winterbottom R, Cunningham DG, Leahy M. A-type cranberry proanthocyanidins and uropathogenic bacterial anti-adhesion activity. Phytochemistry 2005;66: 2281-2291.

[68] Hull RA, Rudy DC, Donovan WH, Wieser IE, Stewart C, Darouiche RO. Virulence properties of Escherichia coli 83972, a prototype strain associated with asymptomatic bacteriuria. Infect Immun 1999;67:429-32.

[69] Itoh Y, Wang X, Hinnebusch BJ, Preston JF, Romeo T. Depolymerization of beta-1,6-N-acetyl-D-glucosamine disrupts the integrity of diverse bacterial biofilms. J Bacteriol 2005;187:382-7.

[70] Izano EA, Sadovskaya I, Vinogradov E, Mulks MH, Velliyagounder K, Ragunath C, et al. Poly-N-acetylglucosamine mediates biofilm formation and antibiotic resistance in Actinobacillus pleuropneumoniae. Microb Pathog 2007;43:1-9.

[71] Izano EA, Amarante MA, Kher WB, Kaplan JB. Differential roles of poly-N-acetylglucosamine surface polysaccharide and extracellular DNA in *Staphylococcus aureus* and *Staphylococcus epidermidis* biofilms. Appl Environ Microbiol 2008;74(2):470-6.

[72] Jackson DW, Suzuki K, Oakford L, Simecka JW, Hart ME, Romeo T. Biofilm formation and dispersal under the influence of the global regulator CsrA of Escherichia coli. J Bacteriol 2002;184:290-301.

[73] Jain P, Parada JP, David A, Smith LG. Overuse of the indwelling urinary tract catheter in hospitalized medical patients. Arch Intern Med 1995;155:1425-9.

[74] Justice SS, Hung C, Theriot JA, Fletcher DA, Anderson GG, Footer MJ, et al. Differentiation and developmental pathways of uropathogenic Escherichia coli in urinary tract pathogenesis. Proc Natl Acad Sci U S A 2004;101:1333-8.

[75] Karatan E, Watnick P. Signals, regulatory networks, and materials that build and break bacterial biofilms. Microbiol Mol Biol Rev 2009;73:310-47.

[76] Kirov SM, Castrisios M, Shaw JG. Aeromonas flagella (polar and lateral) are enterocyte adhesins that contribute to biofilm formation on surfaces. Infect Immun 2004;72:1939-45.

[77] Klevens RM, Edwards JR, Richards CL, Horan TC, Gaynes RP, Pollock DA, et al. Estimating health care-associated infections and deaths in U.S. hospitals, 2002. Public Health Rep 2007;122:160-6.

[78] Klumpp DJ, Weiser AC, Sengupta S, Forrestal SG, Batler RA, Schaeffer AJ. Uropathogenic Escherichia coli potentiates type 1 pilus-induced apoptosis by suppressing NF-kappaB. Infect Immun 2001;69:6689-95.

[79] Kowalczuk D, Ginalska G, Golus J. Characterization of the developed antimicrobial urological catheters. Int J Pharm 2010;402:175-83.

[80] Langermann S, Möllby R, Burlein JE, Palaszynski SR, Auguste CG, DeFusco A, et al. Vaccination with FimH adhesin protects cynomolgus monkeys from colonization and infection by uropathogenic Escherichia coli. J Infect Dis 2000;181:774-8.

[81] Langermann S, Palaszynski S, Barnhart M, Auguste G, Pinkner JS, Burlein J, et al. Prevention of mucosal Escherichia coli infection by FimH-adhesin-based systemic vaccination. Science 1997;276:607-11.

[82] Lasa I, Penadés JR. Bap: a family of surface proteins involved in biofilm formation. Res Microbiol 2006;157:99-107.

[83] Lauriano CM, Ghosh C, Correa NE, Klose KE. The sodium-driven flagellar motor controls exopolysaccharide expression in Vibrio cholerae. J Bacteriol 2004;186:4864-74.

[84] Lellouche J, Kahana E, Elias S, Gedanken A, Banin E. Antibiofilm activity of nanosized magnesium fluoride. Biomaterials 2009;30:5969-78.

[85] Lemon KP, Higgins DE, Kolter R. Flagellar motility is critical for Listeria monocytogenes biofilm formation. J Bacteriol 2007;189:4418-24.

[86] Li X, Zhao H, Lockatell CV, Drachenberg CB, Johnson DE, Mobley HL. Visualization of *Proteus mirabilis* within the matrix of urease-induced bladder stones during experimental urinary tract infection. Infect Immun 2002;70:389-94.

[87] Litwin MS, Saigal CS, Yano EM, Avila C, Geschwind SA, Hanley JM. Urologic diseases in America project: analytical methods and principal findings. J. Urol 2005;173:933-937.

[88] Liu Y, Black MA, Caron L, Camesano TA. Role of cranberry juice on molecular-scale surface characteristics and adhesion behavior of *Escherichia coli*. Biotechnol Bioeng 2006;93:297-305.

[89] Lo E, Nicolle L, Classen D, Arias KM, Podgorny K, Anderson DJ, et al. Strategies to prevent catheter-associated urinary tract infections in acute care hospitals. Infect Control Hosp Epidemiol 2008;29 Suppl 1:S41-50.

[90] Lyte M, Freestone PP, Neal CP, Olson BA, Haigh RD, Bayston R, et al. Stimulation of Staphylococcus epidermidis growth and biofilm formation by catecholamine inotropes. Lancet 2003;361:130-5.

[91] Maki DG, Tambyah PA. Engineering out the risk for infection with urinary catheters. Emerg Infect Dis 2001;7:342-7.

[92] Manefield M, de Nys R, Kumar N, Read R, Givskov M, Steinberg P, et al. Evidence that halogenated furanones from Delisea pulchra inhibit acylated homoserine lactone (AHL)-mediated gene expression by displacing the AHL signal from its receptor protein. Microbiology 1999;145 (Pt 2):283-91.

[93] Marrs CF, Zhang L, Foxman B. Escherichia coli mediated urinary tract infections: are there distinct uropathogenic E. coli (UPEC) pathotypes? FEMS Microbiol Lett 2005;252:183-90.

[94] Marshall KC. Interfaces in microbial ecology. Cambridge, MA: Harvard University Press, 1976. 156 p.

[95] Matsukawa M, Greenberg EP. Putative exopolysaccharide synthesis genes influence Pseudomonas aeruginosa biofilm development. J Bacteriol 2004;186:4449-56.

[96] Matsumura Y, Yoshikata K, Kunisaki S, Tsuchido T. Mode of bactericidal action of silver zeolite and its comparison with that of silver nitrate. Appl Environ Microbiol 2003;69:4278-81.

[97] Mattelaer JJ, Billiet I. Catheters and sounds: the history of bladder catheterisation. Paraplegia 1995;33:429-33.

[98] Morris NS, Stickler DJ. The effect of urease inhibitors on the encrustation of urethral catheters. Urol Res 1998;26:275-9.

[99] Mulvey MA, Lopez-Boado YS, Wilson CL, Roth R, Parks WC, Heuser J, et al. Induction and evasion of host defenses by type 1-piliated uropathogenic Escherichia coli. Science 1998;282:1494-7.

[100] Mulvey MA, Schilling JD, Hultgren SJ. Establishment of a persistent Escherichia coli reservoir during the acute phase of a bladder infection. Infect Immun 2001;69:4572-9.

[101] Munasinghe RL, Yazdani H, Siddique M, Hafeez W. Appropriateness of use of indwelling urinary catheters in patients admitted to the medical service. Infect Control Hosp Epidemiol 2001;22:647-9.

[102] National Nosocomial Infections Surveillance (NNIS) System Report, data summary from January 1992 through June 2004, issued October 2004. Am J Infect Control 2004;32:470-85.

[103] Nickel JC, Downey JA, Costerton JW. Ultrastructural study of microbiologic colonization of urinary catheters. Urology 1989;34:284-91.

[104] Nickel JC, Gristina AG, Costerton JW. Electron microscopic study of an infected Foley catheter. Can J Surg 1985;28:50-1, 4.

[105] Nickel JC, Olson ME, Barabas A, Benediktsson H, Dasgupta MK, Costerton JW. Pathogenesis of chronic bacterial prostatitis in an animal model. Br J Urol 1990;66:47-54.

[106] Nickel JC, Olson M, McLean RJ, Grant SK, Costerton JW. An ecological study of infected urinary stone genesis in an animal model. Br J Urol 1987;59:21-30.

[107] Nicolle LE. Infection control in acute care facilities: Evidence-based patient safety. Can J Infect Dis. 2001;12(3):131-2.

[108] Nicolle LE. Catheter-related urinary tract infection. Drugs Aging 2005;22:627-39.

[109] Oelschlaeger TA, Dobrindt U, Hacker J. Virulence factors of uropathogens. Curr Opin Urol 2002;12:33-8.

[110] Ofek I, Godhar J, Zafriri D, Lis H, Adar R, Sharon N. Anti-*Escherichia coli* adhesion activity of cranberry and blueberry juices. N Engl J Med 1991; 324:1599.

[111] Ohkawa M, Sugata T, Sawaki M, Nakashima T, Fuse H, Hisazumi H. Bacterial and crystal adherence to the surfaces of indwelling urethral catheters. J Urol 1990;143:717-21.

[112] Ohnishi R, Ito H, Kasajima N, Kaneda M, Kariyama R, Kumon H, Hatano T, Yoshida T. Urinary excretion of anthocyanins in humans after cranberry juice ingestion. Biosci Biotechnol Biochem 2006; 70:1681-1687.

[113] Pak J, Pu Y, Zhang ZT, Hasty DL, Wu XR. Tamm-Horsfall protein binds to type 1 fimbriated Escherichia coli and prevents E. coli from binding to uroplakin Ia and Ib receptors. J Biol Chem 2001;276:9924-30.

[114] Parise G, Mishra M, Itoh Y, Romeo T, Deora R. Role of a putative polysaccharide locus in Bordetella biofilm development. J Bacteriol 2007;189:750-60.

[115] Park JH, Cho YW, Cho YH, Choi JM, Shin HJ, Bae YH, et al. Norfloxacin-releasing urethral catheter for long-term catheterization. J Biomater Sci Polym Ed 2003;14:951-62.

[116] Park JH, Cho YW, Kwon IC, Jeong SY, Bae YH. Assessment of PEO/PTMO multiblock copolymer/segmented polyurethane blends as coating materials for urinary catheters: in vitro bacterial adhesion and encrustation behavior. Biomaterials 2002;23:3991-4000.

[117] Pérez-López FR, Haya J, Chedraui P. *Vaccinium macrocarpon*: an interesting option for women with recurrent urinary tract infections and other health benefits. J Obstet Gynaecol Res 2009;35:630-639.

[118] Platt R, Polk BF, Murdock B, Rosner B. Reduction of mortality associated with nosocomial urinary tract infection. Lancet 1983;1:893-7.

[119] Poovendran P, Vidhya N, Murugan S. Antimicrobial Activity of *Coccinia grandis* Against Biofilm and ESBL Producing Uropathogenic *E. coli.* Global J Pharmacol 2011; 5 (1): 23-26.

[120] Pratt LA, Kolter R. Genetic analysis of Escherichia coli biofilm formation: roles of flagella, motility, chemotaxis and type I pili. Mol Microbiol 1998;30:285-93.

[121] Pugach JL, DiTizio V, Mittelman MW, Bruce AW, DiCosmo F, Khoury AE. Antibiotic hydrogel coated Foley catheters for prevention of urinary tract infection in a rabbit model. J Urol 1999;162:883-7.

[122] Regev-Shoshani G, Ko M, Crowe A, Av-Gay Y. Comparative efficacy of commercially available and emerging antimicrobial urinary catheters against bacteriuria caused by E. coli in vitro. Urology 2011;78:334-9.

[123] Regev-Shoshani G, Ko M, Miller C, Av-Gay Y. Slow release of nitric oxide from charged catheters and its effect on biofilm formation by Escherichia coli. Antimicrob Agents Chemother 2010;54:273-9.

[124] Reysenbach AL, Cady SL. Microbiology of ancient and modern hydrothermal systems. Trends Microbiol 2001;9:79-86.

[125] Richards MJ, Edwards JR, Culver DH, Gaynes RP. Nosocomial infections in medical intensive care units in the United States. National Nosocomial Infections Surveillance System. Crit Care Med 1999;27:887-92.

[126] Rijavec M, Starcic Erjavec M, Ambrozic Avgustin J, Reissbrodt R, Fruth A, Krizan-Hergouth V, Zgur-Bertok D. High prevalence of multidrug resistance and random distribution of mobile genetic elements among uropathogenic *Escherichia coli* (UPEC) of the four major phylogenetic groups. Curr Microbiol 2006;53(2):158-62.

[127] Ronald A, Ludwig E. Urinary tract infections in adults with diabetes. Int J Antimicrob Agents 2001;17:287-92.

[128] Ronald A. The etiology of urinary tract infection: traditional and emerging pathogens. Am J Med. 2002;113 Suppl 1A:14S-19S.

[129] Rosen DA, Hooton TM, Stamm WE, Humphrey PA, Hultgren SJ. Detection of intracellular bacterial communities in human urinary tract infection. PLoS Med 2007;4:e329.

[130] Ruben FL, Dearwater SR, Norden CW, Kuller LH, Gartner K, Shalley A, et al. Clinical infections in the noninstitutionalized geriatric age group: methods utilized and incidence of infections. The Pittsburgh Good Health Study. Am J Epidemiol 1995;141:145-57.

[131] Saint S, Elmore JG, Sullivan SD, Emerson SS, Koepsell TD. The efficacy of silver alloy-coated urinary catheters in preventing urinary tract infection: a meta-analysis. Am J Med 1998;105:236-41.

[132] Scott II RD. 2009. The direct medical costs of healthcare associated infections in US hospitals and the benefits of their prevention. http://www.cdc.gov/HAI/pdfs/hai/Scott_CostPaper.pdf

[133] Schumm K, Lam TB. Types of urethral catheters for management of short-term voiding problems in hospitalized adults: a short version Cochrane review. Neurourol Urodyn 2008;27:738-46.

[134] Seeram NP. Berry fruits for cancer prevention: current status and future prospects. J Agric Food Chem 2008; 56:630-635.

[135] Sherlock O, Schembri MA, Reisner A, Klemm P. Novel roles for the AIDA adhesin from diarrheagenic Escherichia coli: cell aggregation and biofilm formation. J Bacteriol 2004;186:8058-65.

[136] Shin JS, Gao Z, Abraham SN. Involvement of cellular caveolae in bacterial entry into mast cells. Science 2000;289:785-8.

[137] Siddiq DM, Darouiche RO. New strategies to prevent catheter-associated urinary tract infections. Nat Rev Urol 2012;9:305-14.

[138] Snyder JA, Lloyd AL, Lockatell CV, Johnson DE, Mobley HL. Role of phase variation of type 1 fimbriae in a uropathogenic Escherichia coli cystitis isolate during urinary tract infection. Infect Immun 2006;74:1387-93.

[139] Sokurenko EV, Chesnokova V, Doyle RJ, Hasty DL. Diversity of the Escherichia coli type 1 fimbrial lectin. Differential binding to mannosides and uroepithelial cells. J Biol Chem 1997;272:17880-6.

[140] Solano C, García B, Valle J, Berasain C, Ghigo JM, Gamazo C, et al. Genetic analysis of Salmonella enteritidis biofilm formation: critical role of cellulose. Mol Microbiol 2002;43:793-808.

[141] Sosa V, Zunino PJ. Effect of *Ibicella lutea* on uropathogenic *Proteus mirabilis* growth, virulence, and biofilm formation. Infect Dev Ctries 2009; 3(10):762-70.

[142] Spiers AJ, Bohannon J, Gehrig SM, Rainey PB. Biofilm formation at the air-liquid interface by the Pseudomonas fluorescens SBW25 wrinkly spreader requires an acetylated form of cellulose. Mol Microbiol 2003;50:15-27.

[143] Srinivasan A, Karchmer T, Richards A, Song X, Perl TM. A prospective trial of a novel, silicone-based, silver-coated Foley catheter for the prevention of nosocomial urinary tract infections. Infect Control Hosp Epidemiol 2006;27:38-43.

[144] Stamm WE, Hooton TM. Management of urinary tract infections in adults. N Engl J Med 1993; 329:1328-1334.

[145] Stark RP, Maki DG. Bacteriuria in the catheterized patient. What quantitative level of bacteriuria is relevant? N Engl J Med 1984;311:560-4.

[146] Stevenson G, Andrianopoulos K, Hobbs M, Reeves PR. Organization of the Escherichia coli K-12 gene cluster responsible for production of the extracellular polysaccharide colanic acid. J Bacteriol 1996;178:4885-93.

[147] Stewart MJ, Parikh S, Xiao G, Tonge PJ, Kisker C. Structural basis and mechanism of enoyl reductase inhibition by triclosan. J Mol Biol 1999;290:859-65.

[148] Stickler DJ. Bacterial biofilms and the encrustation of urethral catheters. *Biofouling 1996;9:*293–305.

[149] Stickler D, Morris N, Moreno MC, Sabbuba N. Studies on the formation of crystalline bacterial biofilms on urethral catheters. Eur J Clin Microbiol Infect Dis 1998;17:649-52.

[150] Stickler D, Young R, Jones G, Sabbuba N, Morris N. Why are Foley catheters so vulnerable to encrustation and blockage by crystalline bacterial biofilm? Urol Res 2003;31:306-11.

[151] Stoodley P, Sauer K, Davies DG, Costerton JW. Biofilms as complex differentiated communities. Annu Rev Microbiol 2002;56:187-209.

[152] Sun TT, Zhao H, Provet J, Aebi U, Wu XR. Formation of asymmetric unit membrane during urothelial differentiation. Mol Biol Rep 1996;23:3-11.

[153] Sun Y, Zeng Q, Zhang Z, Xu C, Wang Y, He J. Decreased urethral mucosal damage and delayed bacterial colonization during short-term urethral catheterization using a novel trefoil urethral catheter profile in rabbits. J Urol 2011;186:1497-501.

[154] Sutherland IW. The biofilm matrix--an immobilized but dynamic microbial environment.. Trends Microbiol 2001;9(5):222-7.

[155] Svanborg C, Bergsten G, Fischer H, Frendéus B, Godaly G, Gustafsson E, et al. The 'innate' host response protects and damages the infected urinary tract. Ann Med 2001;33:563-70.

[156] Tambyah PA. Catheter-associated urinary tract infections: diagnosis and prophylaxis. Int J Antimicrob Agents 2004;24 Suppl 1:S44-8.

[157] Tabibian JH, Gornbein J, Heidari A, Dien SL, Lau VH, Chahal P, Churchill BM, Haake DA. Uropathogens and host characteristics. J Clin Microbiol 2008; 46:3980-3986.

[158] Tambyah PA, Halvorson KT, Maki DG. A prospective study of pathogenesis of catheter-associated urinary tract infections. Mayo Clin Proc 1999;74:131-6.

[159] Tao Y, Pinzón-Arango PA, Howell AB, Camesano TA. Oral consumption of cranberry juice cocktail inhibits molecular-scale adhesion of clinical uropathogenic *Escherichia coli*. J Med Food 2011;14(7-8):739-45.

[160] Taylor CD, Wirsen CO, Gaill F. Rapid microbial production of filamentous sulfur mats at hydrothermal vents. Appl Environ Microbiol 1999;65:2253-5.

[161] Tenke P, Kovacs B, Jäckel M, Nagy E. The role of biofilm infection in urology. World J Urol 2006;24:13-20.

[162] Tenke P, Köves B, Nagy K, Hultgren SJ, Mendling W, Wullt B, et al. Update on biofilm infections in the urinary tract. World J Urol 2012;30:51-7.

[163] Tielker D, Hacker S, Loris R, Strathmann M, Wingender J, Wilhelm S, et al. Pseudomonas aeruginosa lectin LecB is located in the outer membrane and is involved in biofilm formation. Microbiology 2005;151:1313-23.

[164] Topal J, Conklin S, Camp K, Morris V, Balcezak T, Herbert P. Prevention of nosocomial catheter-associated urinary tract infections through computerized feedback to physicians and a nurse-directed protocol. Am J Med Qual 2005;20:121-6.

[165] Toutain CM, Caizza NC, Zegans ME, O'Toole GA. Roles for flagellar stators in biofilm formation by Pseudomonas aeruginosa. Res Microbiol 2007;158:471-7.

[166] Trautner BW, Darouiche RO. Catheter-associated infections: pathogenesis affects prevention. Arch Intern Med 2004a;164:842-50.

[167] Trautner BW, Darouiche RO. Role of biofilm in catheter-associated urinary tract infection. Am J Infect Control 2004b;32:177-83.

[168] Trautner BW, Hull RA, Thornby JI, Darouiche RO. Coating urinary catheters with an avirulent strain of Escherichia coli as a means to establish asymptomatic colonization. Infect Control Hosp Epidemiol 2007;28:92-4.

[169] Tunney MM, Gorman SP. Evaluation of a poly(vinyl pyrollidone)-coated biomaterial for urological use. Biomaterials 2002;23:4601-8.

[170] Umscheid CA, Mitchell MD, Doshi JA, Agarwal R, Williams K, Brennan PJ. Estimating the proportion of healthcare-associated infections that are reasonably preventable and the related mortality and costs. Infect Control Hosp Epidemiol 2011;32:101-14.

[171] van Schaik EJ, Giltner CL, Audette GF, Keizer DW, Bautista DL, Slupsky CM, et al. DNA binding: a novel function of Pseudomonas aeruginosa type IV pili. J Bacteriol 2005;187:1455-64.

[172] Vuong C, Kocianova S, Voyich JM, Yao Y, Fischer ER, DeLeo FR, et al. A crucial role for exopolysaccharide modification in bacterial biofilm formation, immune evasion, and virulence. J Biol Chem 2004;279:54881-6.

[173] Wang X, Preston JF, Romeo T. The pgaABCD locus of Escherichia coli promotes the synthesis of a polysaccharide adhesin required for biofilm formation. J Bacteriol 2004;186:2724-34.

[174] Warren JW. Catheter-associated urinary tract infections. Infect Dis Clin North Am 1997;11:609-22.

[175] Warren JW. Catheter-associated urinary tract infections. Int J Antimicrob Agents 2001;17:299-303.

[176] Watnick PI, Lauriano CM, Klose KE, Croal L, Kolter R. The absence of a flagellum leads to altered colony morphology, biofilm development and virulence in Vibrio cholerae O139. Mol Microbiol 2001;39:223-35.

[177] Whitchurch CB, Tolker-Nielsen T, Ragas PC, Mattick JS. Extracellular DNA required for bacterial biofilm formation. Science 2002; 295(5559):1487.

[178] Wollenweber E. Occurrence of flavonoid aglycones in medicinal plants. Prog Clin Biol Res 1988; 280: 45-55.

[179] Yamamoto S, Tsukamoto T, Terai A, Kurazono H, Takeda Y, Yoshida O. Distribution of virulence factors in *Escherichia coli* isolated from urine of cystitis patients. Microbiol Immunol 1995;39:401-4.

[180] Zhou G, Mo WJ, Sebbel P, Min G, Neubert TA, Glockshuber R, et al. Uroplakin Ia is the urothelial receptor for uropathogenic *Escherichia coli*: evidence from in vitro FimH binding. J Cell Sci 2001;114:4095-103.

[181] Zogaj X, Bokranz W, Nimtz M, Römling U. Production of cellulose and curli fimbriae by members of the family *Enterobacteriaceae* isolated from the human gastrointestinal tract. Infect Immun 2003;71:4151-8.

[182] Zogaj X, Nimtz M, Rohde M, Bokranz W, Römling U. The multicellular morphotypes of *Salmonella* typhimurium and *Escherichia coli* produce cellulose as the second component of the extracellular matrix. Mol Microbiol 2001;39:1452-63.

Section 2

New Aspects in Pediatric Urinary Tract Infections

Chapter 5

Developments Regarding Dysfunctional Voiding and Urinary Tract Infections in Children

Yusuf Kibar and Faysal Gok

Additional information is available at the end of the chapter

http://dx.doi.org/10.5772/53569

1. Introduction

Urinary tract infection (UTI) is the most commonly diagnosed bacterial infections of childhood, and have a significant healthcare impact. Renal parenchymal infection and scarring are well-established complications of UTI in children and can lead to renal insufficiency, hypertension and renal failure. Although frequently encountered and well researched, diagnosis and management of UTI continue to be a controversial issue with many challenges for the clinician [1].

Dysfunctional voiding (DV) imposes a considerable social, developmental and physical burden on children and their families. Children that suffer from DV generally present with complaints of UTI, incontinence, constipation and voiding symptoms such as urinary urgency and frequency. Vesicoureteral reflux (VUR) may also be present in some children with more severe DV, possibly resulting in hydronephrosis, pyelonephritis and even secondary chronic renal insufficiency [2].

The true estimate of DV in the general population is not known. Reported population estimates of DV are based on questionable methodology. A wide variation from 4.2-46.4% has been reported depending on the definition used and the methodology adopted [3, 4]. It is probable that these figures represent a gross overestimate of the actual prevalence. In tertiary care centres, DV constitutes up to 40% of referrals in the Paediatric Urology department [2, 5].

This chapter will focus on the epidemiology, diagnosis and management of DV and UTI in neurologically and anatomically normal children. The discussion will highlight recent developments and research in the clinical approach of DV and UTI.

2. Definitions and classification

Children with significant lower urinary tract symptoms without associated neurological or anatomical abnormalities are considered to have non-neurogenic (idiopathic) lower urinary tract dysfunction (LUTD). It represents a disturbance of the lower urinary tract dynamics affecting urine storage or emptying and can simply be categorized into two types in children [2, 6]:

1. Problems related to the filling (storage) phase include overactive bladder (OAB) syndrome, functional urinary incontinence, and giggle incontinence.
2. Disturbances of the emptying (voiding) phase include dysfunctional voiding (DV), lazy bladder syndrome, Hinman syndrome, and post-void dribbling.

Confusion can occur in identifying these syndromes as they may exist as a single entity or in combination and can be progressive.

Overactive bladder (OAB) syndrome, which is the most common pattern in children with LUTD, includes involuntary detrusor contractions and urethral instability. In children, OAB is the result of sudden and overwhelming urge to void that requires immediate urethral compression by the pelvic floor or by external manoeuvres such as the Vincent curtsy. This syndrome may also result in constipation from chronic pelvic musculature contraction [2]. OAB is thought to be due to a delay in acquisition of cortical inhibition over uninhibited detrusor contractions in the course of achieving the mature voiding pattern of adulthood. Abnormal overactivity of the pelvic floor musculature during voiding, instead of a complete relaxation, results in interrupted micturation [7]. The diagnosis of OAB syndrome can be made on examining the history of incontinence related to urgency, and does not require urodynamic evidence of uninhibited detrusor activity.

Functional urinary incontinence is the failure of the sphincteric mechanism to maintain continence in anatomically normal children. True stress urinary incontinence in which there is an anatomic insufficiency of the sphincteric mechanism to hold urine in transmission of abdominal pressures to the bladder is rare in children [2].

Giggle incontinence is almost exclusively seen in girls and is characterized by large-volume voiding that can occur with laughing. These patients have no voiding symptoms between episodes and no other episodes of incontinence. The diagnosis is based on history alone and, unless there is a history of UTI, no further evaluation is needed. Although the aetiology is not clear, this may be a centrally mediated disorder similar to another disorder, cataplexy, in which an emotional event causes muscle hypotonia. Accordingly, there is evidence that the central nervous system stimulant, methylphenidate, may be effective in prevention of these events [8].

Dysfunctional voiding is an abnormal contraction of the voluntary sphincter and pelvic floor during voiding that is thought to be an acquired disorder that may progress to complete loss of bladder function [9]. Voiding dysfunction has been used and is no longer an acceptable term. This term describes malfunction during the voiding phase only.

http://dx.doi.org/10.5772/53569

It says nothing about the storage phase. The term cannot be applied unless repeat uroflow measurements show curves with a staccato pattern or unless verified by invasive urodynamic investigation [10]. Due to the abnormal contraction of the pelvic floor (pelvic floor dysfunction), constipation is common in these children. Dysfunctional elimination syndrome (DES) is often used to describe this disorder because this term accounts for the link between the difficulty in voiding and defecation caused by the abnormal contraction of the pelvic floor [3]. In recent studies, the rate of OAB in children with LUTD was reported variously as 58% and 71%. It has been suggested that the rate of DV is lower than that of OAB [11, 12].

Lazy bladder syndrome or myogenic failure is the loss of detrusor activity that requires the Valsalva maneuver to fully empty the bladder [2]. This condition is seen in about 7% of all dysfunctional voiders and typically occurs in females with a ratio of 5:1 to males [8]. Long-term fractionated voiding is thought to be the cause of this syndrome in which long voiding times result in loss of the normal detrusor function. Voiding is accomplished by increasing abdominal pressure to empty. Infrequent voids, large-volume post-void residuals with overflow incontinence, and UTIs are the prevalent symptoms and signs. As a rule, urodynamic evaluation demonstrates a large-capacity, very compliant bladder; however, some of these patients may also demonstrate a degree of detrusor overactivity [8].

Hinman syndrome or nonneurogenic neurogenic bladder (NNNB) is often interchanged with occult neuropathic bladder and represents full decompensation of the voiding mechanism. Children will present with day and night-time incontinence, chronic UTIs, and chronic constipation. Urodynamic studies will often show uninhibited detrusor activity during filling, high filling pressures, large post-void residual (PVR) volumes, and abnormal activity of the pelvic floor musculature during voiding. Imaging studies results are frequently abnormal with hydroureteronephrosis secondary to VUR being common [2].

Post-void dribbling is a disorder in which incontinence of urine occurs immediately after micturition. This syndrome is more common in female patients and is thought to be secondary to retained urine in the vagina that leaks after standing. Even though it is more likely to occur in obese girls it can also happen frequently in girls who are thin. This pattern can be seen on voiding cystourethrography. This can produce irritation of the labia, dysuria as the urine passes over the irritated skin, a reduced desire to void, incomplete emptying, and eventually recurrent UTI with its consequent changes in bladder function that further aggravate the clinical picture. Although these symptoms usually resolve with age and normal growth, the child may improve the symptoms more abruptly by facing backwards on the toilet with her body tilted forward and her legs straddling the toilet, or by manually spreading the labia majora with fingers as she voids [8].

3. Aetiology and pathogenesis

The aetiology of DV in otherwise healthy, neurologically intact children remains a matter of debate. In the absence of any neurologic or anatomic findings, the voiding patterns in DV are often believed to originate from behavioural issues. These behavioural traits may evolve from adverse events that occur around or after the time of toilet training and/or personal stresses [13]. Severe emotional stressors, such as sexual abuse mainly in girls, has been associated with DV, and should be considered in a child, especially a girl, who presents with new onset DV and no other identifiable etiologic factor [4, 5].

Detrusor overactivity as a component of DV may represent a persistence of the normal infant voiding pattern after toilet training. It may be that a mild delay in the maturation of the central nervous system disrupts the ability of these children to learn true voluntary control over the micturition reflex [5, 14]. An alternative theory to the development of the urge syndrome hypothesizes that detrusor overactivity is caused by the transient obstruction that occurs with DV [15]. In support of the belief that the roots of DV may be grounded in behavioural issues or central nervous system developmental delays, an association has been demonstrated between DV and attention deficit hyperactivity disorder (ADHD). Higher rates of enuresis, urinary incontinence, constipation, and other voiding symptoms have been described in children with ADHD [16, 17].

As a result of studies of DV diagnosed in infancy, a congenital or genetic component to the disorder has also been postulated. Small series of infants with signs and symptoms consistent with NNNB syndromes have been reported [18, 19]. Furthermore, DV has been linked to the Ochoa syndrome, a genetic disorder with an autosomal recessive inheritance pattern. The gene locus at chromosome 10q23-q24 is identified as the defective gene in Ochoa syndrome. It is postulated to be the possible gene locus of the NNNB described by Hinman and Allan [20]. This information casts doubt on the commonly held belief that disturbance of behaviour is the sole cause of NNNB because these findings are present at or near the time of birth.

At least some patients with DV represent occult neurogenic problems that will manifest provided these patients are followed longitudinally [21]. In all individuals with unexplained severe DV, search for an unidentified neurological lesion must be made. A subtle neurological insult could present as DV. Such lesions may or may not be detectable with current imaging technologies. Routine magnetic resonance imaging in children with lower urinary tract problems without overt neurological signs and symptoms has a low yield of 7.5% but this may be improved by targeting children with abnormal cutaneous findings [22]. Tethered cord syndrome may be identified in some patients with subtle neurological signs and symptoms. Classical tethered cord has been diagnosed on the basis of pathologically elongated conus or conus that lies below the L2 level. However, anecdotal successful outcomes following surgical division of the filum in children with apparently normally located cords suggest that the cord may sometimes be abnormally stretched without being at an abnormal location [23]. Such subtle lesions might also explain the occasional presentation in infancy when the problem has its onset before toilet training has commenced [19]. Surgical division of the filum terminale in such patients is controversial but may yield improvements in bladder dysfunction [24].

Another possible indirect evidence for an unidentified neurological lesion in these patients is the association of a peculiar facial expression in some children with DV [25].

The association of facial expression with bladder function in this "Urofacial Syndrome" has been explained by the proximity of the cortical centres for the bladder and facial expression in the brain. Presumably, this makes an association of abnormality between the two centres more likely.

A higher than expected association of idiopathic hypercalciuria, ranging from 21-30%, has been noted in children with DV syndromes. However, almost all responded to behavioural therapy, dietary modifications and anticholinergics and treatment specifically directed at hypercalciuria were needed in only two percent [26]. The reason for an association between hypercalciuria and DV remains unclear. The authors postulated that calcium microcrystallization may cause injury to the urothelium and this could trigger a variety of urinary symptoms including DV.

It is probable that the entity DV is not homogenous and that there are several distinct aetiologies that can lead to it. The end result is one of a dyssynergic sphincteric activity in the absence of a clearly defined neurological reason.

4. Association of LUTD with UTI and VUR

There is not sufficient reported data on the relationship between the type of LUTD with UTI and VUR. The earliest studies of LUTD mostly dealt with either OAB or DV. This is a somewhat artificial distinction, as these conditions are often combined and sometimes difficult to separate. For that reasons this association will be presented in LUTD children as a whole.

The association between LUTD and UTI has been established, though the causal relationship is not clear. Recurrent UTI has been shown in any studies to be higher in VUR patients with LUTD than in those without such dysfunction [3, 27, 28]. It has been demonstrated that adequate management of LUTD not only decreases the rate of UTI but also increases resolution of the VUR [27, 29]. Traditionally, recurrent UTI and pyelonephritis have been recognized as potential causes of permanent renal damage [30]. Current opinion is that VUR alone is not sufficient to cause UTI or renal damage. Holland et al. reported that girls with primary VUR followed up for 10 years, with no recurrent UTI, did not develop renal scars [31]. Linshaw showed that VUR does not threaten the kidney as long as UTI is promptly treated [32]. The results of these studies suggest that the association between VUR and UTI is necessary for renal damage to occur, mainly in situations of low detrusor pressure. However, VUR may predispose invasion of the renal parenchyma by bacteria. It has been reported that LUTD is an important risk factor for VUR and renal damage [33]. In addition, current studies have showed that increased intravesical pressure associated with LUTD is a primary factor for inducing reflux and renal damage [12, 34]. In patients who had UTI the presence of reflux increased the rate of renal damage [12].

VUR in LUTD is theorized to be not the result of a short mucosal tunnel, but to be the consequence of the high filling and voiding pressures. In patients with LUTD, uninhibited detrusor contractions and voluntary constriction of the sphincter, causing a functional obstruction, increase the intravesical pressure. Increased intravesical pressure can promote VUR through a possible marginal competence in the valve mechanism [34, 35]. Recent studies have shown that the prevalence of VUR among children with idiopathic LUTD is between 14% and 46% [11, 12]. Some reports have emphasized bilateral reflux associated with LUTD [12, 36].

Van Gool et al. addressed the relationship between DV and reflux for the first time with a retrospective questionnaire in 1992 [37]. The prevalence of uncoordination between the detrusor and urethral sphincter approached 18% and included voiding pattern abnormalities such as urge syndrome, staccato voiding, fractionated and incomplete voiding, and voiding postponement. They also found that, in those children who had spontaneous resolution of their VUR, there was a lower prevalence of DV.

It is important to carefully assess all children with reflux for subtle signs of DV. Children with DV are more likely to have recurrent UTIs, have mild bilateral reflux with less spontaneous resolution, and are less likely to have success with surgical management. The treatment of DV in such children can improve the chances of spontaneous resolution of the reflux and may also reduce recurrent urinary infection. Koff et al. [3] reported on their series of children with VUR, who either resolved spontaneously or were surgically treated, and found that DES was observed in 43% of children with primary VUR and in 77% of a subset of these children who had breakthrough UTI. The presence of DES patterns was associated with a longer time for spontaneous resolution of low-grade reflux and with unsuccessful surgical outcomes. Of children in the surgically treated group, only those with DES developed recurrent and/or contralateral reflux. Children with untreated DV undergoing ureteral re-implantation may be at a higher risk for developing recurrent reflux or a new bladder diverticulum [38].

Contrary to these results, Chen and colleagues reported that VUR and UTI are not independent of DV [39]. Their findings are new observations contradicting the previous belief that both UTI and VUR are independently associated with DES. Chen et al. performed a multivariate analysis on 2759 paediatric urology patients, further examining the relationship between DES, VUR, and UTI. Their data demonstrated a higher rate of DES in girls than in boys: 43.7% compared with 23.8%. This group also found that there was no difference in the presence of DES in patients with unilateral and bilateral VUR. Surprisingly, they observed no association of VUR or UTI individually with DES but rather DES was only noted when both of these issues were present. Although this large-scale multivariate analysis is a more statistically powerful study than previous smaller retrospective analyses, the data could be potentially skewed in that all of the patients were recruited from a paediatric urology population, which is not representative of the general paediatric population. Patients with known reflux could potentially be protected from DES by prophylactic antibiotics or continued clinical follow-up in a specialty setting. On the other hand, it is suggested that there may be two types of reflux: one that is primary or congenital in nature and another that is secondary and in part due to DES and UTI. This study is in line with the neuroplastic theory that postulates that hypertrophy of the bladder and bowel musculature is caused by trophic factors released during pelvic floor hyperactivity secondary to central nervous disturbances [40]. Hypertrophy can lead to an increase in risk factors that predispose the urinary tract to more UTIs and more severe VUR including anatomic bladder abnormalities, constipation, increased residual urine, higher voiding pressures, and increased urethral bacteria colonization secondary to turbulent flow [41, 42]. Turbulent flow is of particular importance as eddy currents formed by nonlaminar flow leads to reflux of periurethral bacteria to the proximal urethra and bladder (milk back phenomenon), causing recurrent infections.

The pelvic floor musculature is closely related to bowel and bladder. Isolated contraction of the pelvic floor musculature was found to lead to spontaneous contraction of the bladder. The cycle of pelvic floor dysfunction contributing to recurrent UTIs and VUR can cause worsening bladder and bowel symptoms, and increased pelvic floor dysfunction with functional obstruction. Eventually this can lead to a hypertrophied, small-capacity bladder with high-pressure voiding that will lead to renal damage. The integral relationship between the pelvic floor activity with UTIs and VUR can be used as a model for developing treatment strategies in affected children to address the cognitive and behavioural aspects of DV and prevent irreversible damage to the upper urinary tract [40].

5. Diagnosis and evaluation

Clinical symptoms may vary from mild incontinence to severe disorders with endpoints of irreversible bladder dysfunction with VUR, UTI and resulting nephropathy [8]. Children with DV voiding often present with urinary incontinence both during the day as well as at night. They may have urinary frequency, urgency, urge incontinence or nocturnal enuresis. Such storage symptoms may result from associated detrusor overactivity, urinary infection or reduced bladder capacity consequent to large residual urine and may be aggravated by constipation or behavioural disorders. A distinctive facial expression may be noted in some of these patients [8].

Diagnosis relies heavily on a good history and physical examination, but also includes radiologic and urodynamic evaluation. The history should be directed towards the identification of children with neurologic or anatomic causes of their symptoms, and then distinguish between which form or pattern of voiding dysfunction is present. Components of this history include maternal medical issues, perinatal history, developmental milestones, scholastic performance, behavioural history, specifics around toilet training, patterns of voiding and bowel movements, history of UTI, and family history of voiding dysfunction. The use of a 3-day voiding diary is often helpful to identify the frequency of voiding, voided volumes, and timing of incontinent episodes [9].

Clinical examination must include an assessment of higher mental functions and their age-appropriateness and basic neurological evaluation. On physical examination, attention should be paid to the back and lower spine for cutaneous manifestations of an occult spinal dysraphism and/or sacral agenesis. Neurologic examination should include assessment of lower extremity function, rectal tone, perineal/anal sensation, and intactness of bulbocavernosus reflex. The external genitalia should also be examined. Bowel function should be evaluated in detail.

Further evaluation of the child with DV continues with a urinalysis and urine culture. The scout film, or plain film of the abdomen (KUB), can be used to assess the spine and sacrum, and for evidence of constipation.

A renal and bladder ultrasonography with a pre-void and post-void image should be obtained to assess for evidence of obstructive uropathy, an ureterocele, bladder wall thickness, and residual urine volume. Studies in healthy infants and toddlers have shown that they do not empty the bladder completely every time but they do so at least once during a 4-hour observation period. In older children, a consistent residual of >20 ml is considered abnormal [29].

The diagnosis of DV in children hinges upon the repeated demonstration of a staccato pattern on uroflowmetry testing. The normal uroflow pattern is a bell-shaped curve with a smooth up-slope and down-slope. OAB may produce an explosive voiding contraction that appears in the flow measurement as a high amplitude curve of short duration, that is, a tower-shaped curve. A child with organic outlet tract obstruction often has low amplitude and rather even flow curve, that is, a plateau-shaped curve. Finally, in case of an underactive or acontractile detrusor when contraction of the abdominal muscles creates the main force for bladder evacuation, the flow curve usually shows discrete peaks corresponding to each strain, separated by segments with zero flow, namely, an interrupted or fractionated flow curve. The staccato pattern of voiding has been considered classical of DV. Sphincter overactivity during voiding is seen as sharp peaks and troughs in the flow curve, which is as an irregular or staccato flow curve [10] (Figure 1). To label flow as staccato, the fluctuations should be more than the square root of the maximum flow rate. When combined with needle or surface EMG, increased striated urethral sphincter-pelvic floor complex activity can be noted [9]. Less invasive uroflowmetry, perineal electromyography, and PVR comprise the preferred modality at our institution for screening and monitoring response to treatment. Before flow study, bladder ultrasonography is used to ensure adequate volume and exclude patients with overdistention of the bladder. Overdistention of the bladder can obscure results, causing an artificial increase in PVR volumes in normal children [43].

There have been efforts to standardize scoring systems in the evaluation of children with DV. These scoring systems would be beneficial in classifying the type and severity of DV to determine necessary treatment modalities. Farhat et al. introduced the Dysfunctional Voiding Scoring System (DVSS) by comparing the scores of the children aged 3-10 years with age-matched controls across 10 questions related to urinary incontinence, voiding habits, urgency, posturing, bowel habits and stressful life conditions [44]. Nine of these questions are scored between 0 and 3 depending on whether the problem is noted almost never (0), less than half the time (1), about half the time (2) or almost every time (3). The last question is addressed to the parents to identify a stress situation in the family. The authors derived cutoff values of 6 and 9 for girls and boys respectively for making a diagnosis of DV. A small prospective cohort was analyzed by Upadhyay and colleagues to determine the validity of the DVSS in children with reflux. A positive correlation between symptom score improvement and resolution of VUR was found [45]. Another scoring system is the "Dysfunctional voiding and incontinence scoring system" and designed by Akbal et al. They reported that the children with a score of 8.5 or greater had voiding abnormalities with 90% sensitivity and 90% specificity [46]. The last one was devised by Afshar et al, *which* was a 14-item 5-point Likert scale questionnaire for children with dysfunctional elimination with a cut-off score of 11 [47]. This questionnaire was valid and reliable for diagnosing dysfunctional elimination syndrome. The validity of these scoring systems has not yet been evaluated in large prospective trials.

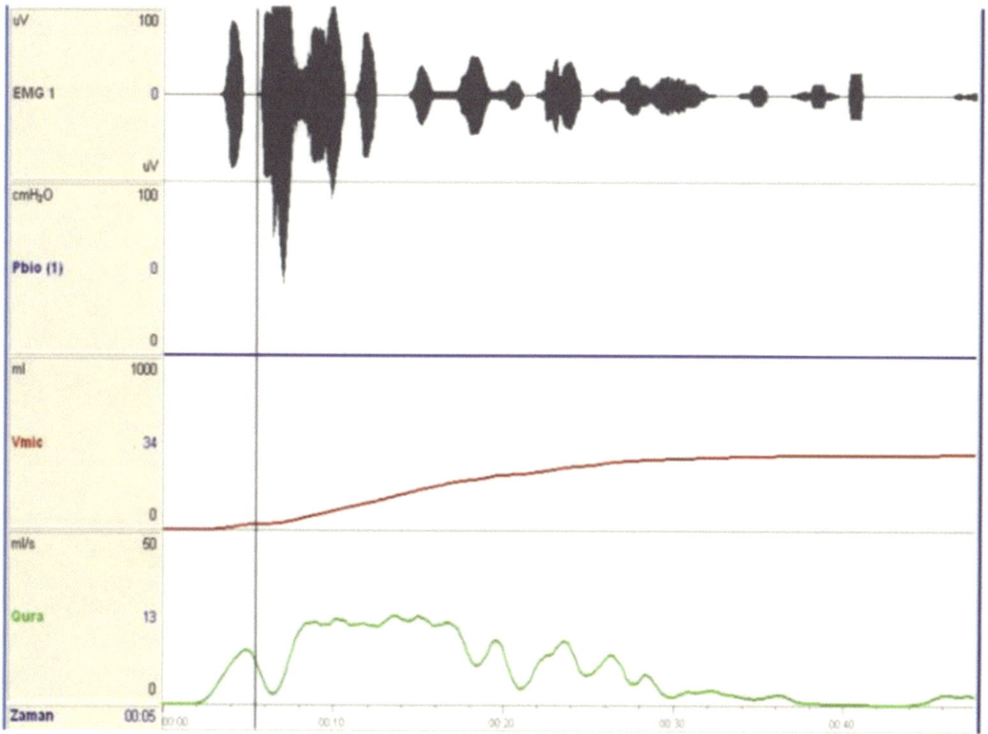

Figure 1. Example of a child with staccato flow and high EMG activity on Uroflow-EMG.

Perineal USG has been used in women with DV to assess sphincter volume [48]. Perineal USG can also be used to evaluate paradoxical pelvic floor movement which may often be seen in children with DV [49]. Abdominal USG has also been used for chronic constipation in children with DV. Rectal diameter greater than 3.5 cm signifies constipation [50].

Children with DV often show abnormalities on voiding cystourethrogram (VCUG). A VCUG may demonstrate VUR, bladder trabeculation, a diverticulum, a large bladder capacity, or a large post-void residual. Girls may exhibit the spinning top urethra during voiding, which results from dilation of the posterior urethra secondary to detrusor-sphincter uncoordination during voiding [51] (Figure 2). Dilatation of the prostatic urethra may be observed in boys. VCUG should be performed when there is a history of recurrent UTI or a febrile UTI, thickened bladder wall on ultrasound, children older than 5 years with day and nighttime incontinence, or children at puberty with persistent enuresis.

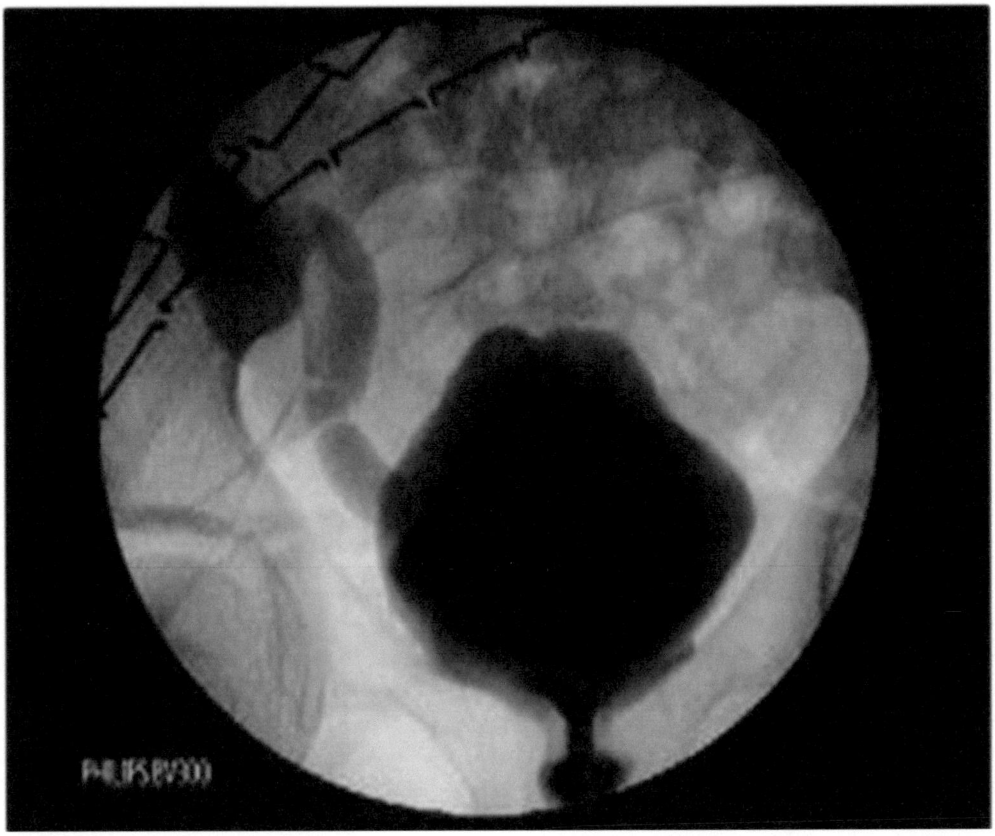

Figure 2. A 6-year old female child with spinning top urethra and right grade 4 VUR on VCUG.

In patients with suspicion of anatomical abnormalities of the lower urinary tract, a diagnostic cystoscopy may be performed. Routine diagnostic cystoscopy is not recommended [52].

Urodynamic evaluation remains an uncomfortable test for children. Cooperation of the child and the narrow size of the urethra are the major hurdles. A relaxed child-friendly environment and patience on the part of the technician are paramount. Full urodynamic studies are considered invasive and should be reserved for children with neurogenic bladder dysfunction, severe DV, myogenic failure, or symptoms that do not improve with therapy [8, 52]. Urodynamic criteria for DV include too large or small bladder capacity, poor bladder compliance, detrusor overactivity or premature contractions, an unsustained voiding contraction, excessive voiding pressure, an intermittent uroflow pattern, or elevated residual urine.

6. Treatment of DV

Urotherapy is the nonsurgical, nonpharmacologic treatment of lower urinary tract function and can be defined as a bladder re-education or rehabilitation program aiming at correction of filling and voiding difficulties. Standard urotherapy is a combination of informing the child and the family about the normal lower urinary tract function and what is abnormal in the patient's voiding and correcting the abnormal voiding habits, lifestyle with regard to fluid intake and diet.

In the setting of discomfort with voiding or dysuria, all efforts should be made to eliminate any dietary irritants, such as caffeine, carbonated beverages, citrus juices, and chocolate. Furthermore, skin care should be initiated in children with eroded or irritated perineal areas from incontinence.

Education emphasizing timed voiding, fluid management, and pelvic floor exercises are key components of the initial management for DV. In addition, education concerning proper posture during voiding should be emphasized to minimize abdominal musculature straining. Proper sitting technique with buttock and foot support and comfortable hip position is necessary to enable voiding without recruitment of the abdominal muscles [53, 54]. Hygiene education is also important to limit local skin inflammation that may contribute to holding maneuvers and DV. In this way, coordinated voiding with a relaxed pelvic floor can be facilitated at the initiation of management.

Treatment of constipation is also important component of the initial management for DV [55]. Fecal impaction must be managed prior to maintenance therapy. For this purpose laxatives, stool softeners, and enemas is recommended. Maintenance with balanced diet, fibre supplementation, and oral medications such as mineral oil, polyethylene glycol and lactulose are recommended to maintain a goal of one bulky bowel movement a day. Treatment of constipation alone has been shown to resolve lower urinary tract abnormalities. Enuresis resolved in 63% and daytime incontinence in 89% of patients presenting with constipation and incontinence in one study [56]. In the same study, resolution of constipation also resolved recurrent UTIs.

Biofeedback therapy is the next line of treatment after conservative approaches have been initiated. Biofeedback is a specific treatment modality that aims to retrain the patient's voiding with the assistance of a computer game. Biofeedback has been used in children as young as four years of age [57]. There is no standard protocol for the correct teaching of biofeedback, but in general there are 2 methods. Real-time uroflowmetry allows the patient to view the urine flow rate that in turn can be used to teach the child to relax his/her pelvic floor musculature with voiding. This method is recommended in children with pelvic floor hyperactivity and no OAB symptoms. Sphincter or pelvic floor electromyography can also be used to teach patients how to voluntarily control their pelvic floor musculature during voiding and thus reduce or prevent detrusor-sphincter incoordination. The advantage in using this method lies in its ability to teach a guarding reflex in addition to the relaxation of the pelvic floor during voiding.

Improvement in incontinence, UTIs, VUR, and constipation with biofeedback therapy is well documented in the literature. Upwards of 80% children will experience improvement marked by a reduction in incontinence and recurrent urinary infection [58] (Figure 3). Factors that have been found to improve efficacy of biofeedback include compliance, normal bladder capacity, number of sessions, and use of animation. Independent risk factors to predict failure identified by Herndon and colleagues are small bladder capacity and compliance to therapy [40]. Results appear durable at three years and the treatment also seems to help those children in whom urotherapy has failed [59]. The inclusion of biofeedback in urotherapy is more likely to lead to an improvement in residual urine [60].

For patients who fail to respond to the above conservative measures, medical therapy is often helpful. Anticholinergic agents serve to decrease detrusor overactivity and increase functional bladder capacity in patients with urge syndrome or a detrusor overactivity. Anticholinergics have been shown to provide effective long-term management of detrusor overactivity and may also contribute to a quicker resolution of VUR in the setting of DV [61, 62].

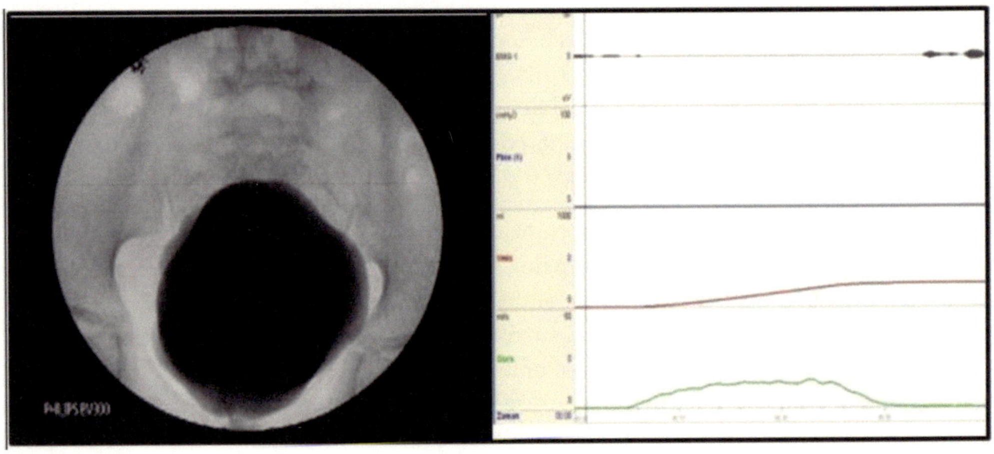

Figure 3. The results of the biofeedback after 4 sessions of treatment in the same child; the appearance of urethra normalized, right grade 4 VUR disappeared on VCUG, and flow curve and EMG activity became normal on Uroflow-EMG.

For patients with small bladder capacity and low PVR in which DV did not improve with 3 sessions of biofeedback, oxybutynin is effective. For children with small capacity bladders and high PVR, a full biofeedback session is often necessary to isolate pelvic floor muscles and lower PVR before initiation of anticholinergics. About 87% of these patients with small-capacity bladders who do not improve with biofeedback will improve with the addition of anticholinergics [40].

Clean intermittent catheterization (CIC) has been shown to be useful in children with high PVR volumes or myogenic failure that do not improve with standard therapy. This therapeutic approach has become routine in many patients with DV of various aetiologies. Pohl et al. [63] described their experience with using CIC in the treatment of dysfunctional voiding with a large post-void residual urine volume. It proved to be well tolerated and allowed patients to rapidly attain continence and eliminate recurrent UTI by achieving more effective bladder emptying.

Alpha-adrenergic blockade of receptors at the bladder neck and urethra results in relaxation of smooth muscle and theoretically enables more complete bladder emptying. Although the results have been somewhat mixed, several studies have shown efficacy in reducing subjective symptoms and improving objective urinary parameters in children with DV and increased PVR [64, 65]. Dramatic improvement in flow, initiation of voiding, and PVR was documented in one study by Donohoe and colleagues [66]. All children that met the criteria of primary bladder neck dysfunction (low flow rate, low EMG activity, and delayed initiation of voiding) improved with alpha-blocker therapy and those that discontinued therapy returned to baseline symptoms.

The transurethral injection of botulinum toxin into the striated urethral sphincter has been beneficial in spinal cord injury patients with detrusor sphincter dyssynergia [67]. Several small studies have demonstrated improvement [68-70]. Botulinum toxin has also been proposed as a potentially new treatment regimen to improve bladder emptying for children with DV who have failed standard therapy. Petronijevic et al examined the role of combined the injection of botulinum toxin-A (BTX-A) and biofeedback in the management of the female children with DV who were refractory to standard therapy, and analyzed their clinical outcomes. The dose of 500 units of BTX-A was diluted in 2.5 ml saline and injected transperineally around the urethral meatus at the 3, 6, 9 and 12 o'clock positions, 1 to 2 cm deep into the external urinary sphincter. After treatment the mean voided volume increased while post-void residual urine volume decreased significantly. Significant differences in other uroflowmetry parameters were not found [71]. In another study, Radojicic et al. investigated the results of BTX-A into the urethral sphincter and/or pelvic floor muscle injection combined with behavioural and biofeedback therapy in children with DV resistant to previous treatments, including behavioural, biofeedback and alpha-blockers in 8 boys and 12 girls. The dose of 100 IU BTX-A was diluted in 4 ml saline and injected by a transperineal 21 or 23 gauge needle in the pelvic floor, including the external sphincter. Six months after treatment residual urine decreased significantly in 17 of 20 patients. Nine patients re-established a normal voiding curve and 8 showed improvement. Three did not manifest any significant improvement [72]. The limitations of the studies advocating the use of botulinum toxin are small sample size, lack of standard dosing, and nonrandomization.

Sacral neuromodulation has been successful in children with refractory DV, but the invasiveness of this modality has limited its use in children without neurologic deficits [73]. Its feasibility and efficacy has been well demonstrated [74]. Storage symptoms resolve in about three-fourths of children [74]. The response of DV to neuromodulation with the Interstim neuromodulation device was modest. In a single centre study, urinary incontinence, urgency and frequency, nocturnal enuresis and constipation were improved or resolved in 88%, 69%, 89%, 69% and 71% of the patients, respectively [74]. In a multi-institutional study, about 60% of children with voiding difficulty had some benefit [75]. Neuromodulation offers the additional incentive of a potential improvement in constipation and irritable bowel symptoms [74, 76].

Less invasive neuromodulatory devices such as tibial nerve stimulation and transcutaneous electrical nerve stimulation (TENS) have been proposed as treatment modalities. Capitanucci et al. evaluated the efficacy of percutaneous tibial nerve stimulation for different types of paediatric LUTD. A total of 14 children with idiopathic OAB, 14 with DV, 5 with underactive bladder, 4 with underactive valve bladder and 7 with neurogenic bladder resistant to conventional therapy underwent percutaneous tibial nerve stimulation weekly for 30 min on a weekly schedule for 12 weeks. Patients with DV were significantly more likely to benefit as compared to those with OAB at rates of up to 100 % [77]. TENS has had success in the treatment of OAB syndrome when compared with placebo in one prospective trial [78]. The use of neuromodulation as treatment modality in refractory LUTD is promising, but larger prospective trials will be necessary to solidify its role as a treatment modality.

Author details

Yusuf Kibar[1*] and Faysal Gok[2]

*Address all correspondence to: ykibar@gata.edu.tr

1 Gulhane Military Medical Academy, Department of Urology, Section of Paediatric Urology, Ankara, Turkey

2 Gulhane Military Medical Academy, Department of Peadiatrics, Division of Paediatric Nephrology, Ankara, Turkey

References

[1] Kibar Y. Current Managenement of Urinary Tract Infection in Children. In: Tenke P. (ed.) Urinary Tract Infections. Rijeka: InTech; 2011. p267-284.

[2] Ballek NK, McKenna PH. Lower urinary tract dysfunction in childhood. Urol Clin N Am 2010;37:215-228.

[3] Koff SA, Wagner TT, Jayanthi VR. The relationship among dysfunctional elimination syndromes, primary vesicoureteral reflux and urinary tract infections in children. J Urol 1998;160:1019-1022.

[4] Ellsworth PI, Merguerian PA, Copening ME. Sexual abuse: another causative factor in dysfunctional voiding. J Urol 1995;153:773-776.

[5] Bauer SB, Retik AB, Colodny AH, Hallett M, Khoshbin S, Dyro FM. The unstable bladder of childhood. Urol Clin North Am 1980;7(2):321-336.

[6] Bauer SB, Yeung CK, Sihoe JD. Voiding dysfunction in children: neurogenic and non-neurogenic. In: Kavoussi LR, Novick AC, Partin AW. (eds.) Campbell's Urology. 9th edition. Philadelphia: WB Saunders Co; 2007. p.3604-55.

[7] Franco I. Overactive bladder in children. Part 1: pathophysiology. J Urol 2007;178(3 Pt 1):761-8.

[8] Feldman AS, Bauer SB. Diagnosis and management of dysfunctional voiding. Curr Opin Pediatr 2006;18:139-147.

[9] Chase J, Austin P, Hoebeke P, McKenna P; International Children's Continence Society. The management of dysfunctional voiding in children: a report from the Standardisation Committee of the International Children's Continence Society. J Urol 2010;183(4):1296-302.

[10] Neveus T, von Gontard A, Hoebeke P, Hjälmas K, Bauer S, Bower W, Jorgensen TM, Rittig S, Walle JV, Yeung CK, Djurhuus JC. The standardization of terminology of lower urinary tract function in children and adolescents: report from the Standardization Committee of the International Children's Continence Society. J Urol 2006;176(1):314-24.

[11] Hoebeke P, Van Laecke E, Van Camp C, Raes A, Van De Walle J. One thousand video-urodynamics studies in children with non-neurogenic bladder sphincter dysfunction. BJU Int 2001;87:575-80.

[12] Ural Z, Ulman I, Avanoglu A. Bladder dynamics and vesicoureteric reflux: factors associated with idiopathic lower urinary tract dysfunction in children. J Urol 2008;179:1564-67.

[13] Bauer SB. Special considerations of the overactive bladder in children. Urology 2002; 60(suppl 5A):43-48.

[14] Koff SA, Solomon MH, Lane GA, Lieding KC. Urodynamic studies in anesthetized children. J Urol 1980;123:61-63.

[15] Bauer SB, Koff SA, Jayanthi VR. Voiding dysfunction in children: neurogenic and non-neurogenic. In: Walsh PC, Retik AB, Vaughn ED, Wein AJ. (eds.) Campbell's Urology. 8th Ed. Philadelphia: WB Saunders Co; 2002. pp.2231-2283.

[16] Bhatia M, Nigam V, Bohra N, Malik S. Attention deficit disorder with hyperactivity among paediatric outpatients. J Child Psychol Psychiatry 1991;32:297-306.

[17] Duel BP, Steinberg-Epstein R, Hill M, Lerner M. A survey of voiding dysfunction in children with attention deficit-hyperactivity disorder. J Urol 2003;170:1521-1524.

[18] Jayanthi VR, Khoury AE, McLorie GA, Churchill BM, Khoury AE. The nonneurogenic neurogenic bladder of early infancy. J Urol 1997;158 (3 Pt 2):1281-5.

[19] Al Mosawi AJ. Identification of nonneurogenic neurogenic bladder in infants. Urology 2007;70(2):355-6.

[20] Ochoa B. Can a congenital dysfunctional bladder be diagnosed from a smile? The Ochoa syndrome updated. Pediatr Nephrol 2004;19(1):6-12.

[21] Carlson KV, Rome S, Nitti VW. Dysfunctional voiding in adult females. J Urol 2001;165:143-7.

[22] Afshar K, Blake T, Jaffari S, MacNeily AE, Poskitt K, Sargent M. Spinal cord magnetic resonance imaging for investigation of nonneurogenic lower urinary tract dysfunction-can the yield be improved? J Urol 2007;178:1748-50.

[23] Tubbs RS, Oakes WJ. Can the conus medullaris in normal position be tethered? Neurol Res 2004;26:727-31.

[24] Steinbok P, Kariyattil R, MacNeily AE. Comparison of section of filum terminale and non-neurosurgical management for urinary incontinence in patients with normal conus position and possible occult tethered cord syndrome. Neurosurgery 2007;61:550-5.

[25] Ochoa B, Gorlin RJ. Urofacial (ochoa) syndrome. Am J Med Genet 1987;27:661-7.

[26] Parekh DJ, Pope JC IV, Adams MC, Brock JW 3rd. The role of hypercalciuria in a subgroup of dysfunctional voiding syndromes of childhood. J Urol 2000;164:1008-10.

[27] Snodgrass W. The impact of treated dysfunctional voiding on the nonsurgical management of vesicoureteric reflux. J Urol 1998;160:1823-5.

[28] Sjostrom S, Sillen U, Bachelard M, Hansson S, Stockland E. Spontaneous resolution of high grade infantile vesicoureteral reflux. J Urol 2004;172:694-8.

[29] Kibar Y, Ors O, Demir E, Kalman S, Sakallioglu O, Dayanc M. Results of biofeedback treatment on reflux resolution rates in children. Urology 2007;70:563-6.

[30] Winberg J. Progressive renal damage from infection with or without reflux. J Urol 1992;148:1733-4.

[31] Holland N, Jackson E, Kazee M, Conrad GR, Ryo UY. Relation of urinary tract infection and vesicoureteral reflux to scars: follow up in 38 patients. J Pediatr 1990;116(5):S65-71.

[32] Linshaw MA. Asymptomatic bacteriuria and vesicoureteral reflux in children. Kidney Int 1996;50:312-29.

[33] Naseer SR, Steinhardt GF. New renal scars in children with urinary tract infection, vesicoureteral reflux and voiding dysfunction: a prospective evaluation. J Urol 1997;158:566-8.

[34] Acar B, Arıkan FI, Germiyanoglu C, Dallar Y. Influence of high bladder pressure on vesicoureteral reflux and its resolution. Urol Int 2009;82:77-80.

[35] Sillen U. Bladder dysfunction and vesicoureteral reflux. Adv Urol 2008;815472:1-8.

[36] Soygur T, Arıkan N, Yesilli C¸ Gogus O. Relationship among pediatric voiding dysfunction and vesicoureteral reflux and renal scars. Urology 1999;54:905-8.

[37] Van Gool JD, Hjalmas K, Tamminen-Mobius T, Olbing H. Historical clues to the complex of dysfunctional voiding, urinary tract infection and vesicoureteral reflux. J Urol 1992; 148(5 Pt 2):1699–1702.

[38] Tilanus M, Klijn A, Dik P, de Kort L, de Jong T. Urodynamic findings and functional or anatomical obstructions in children who developed bladder diverticula after reimplantation of the ureter. Neurourol Urodyn 2009;28:241-5.

[39] Chen JJ, Mao W, Homayoon K, Steinhardt GF. A multivariate analysis of dysfunctional elimination syndrome and its relationships with gender, urinary tract infection and vesicoureteral reflux in children. J Urol 2004;171:1907-10.

[40] Herndon CDA, Decambre M, McKenna PH. Changing concepts concerning the management of vesicoureteral reflux. J Urol 2001;166:1439-43.

[41] Whelan CM, McKenna PH. Dysfunctional voiding as a co-factor of recurrent UTI. Contemp Urol 2004;16:58-73.

[42] Hinman F. Mechanisms for the entry of bacteria and the establishment of urinary infection in female children. J Urol 1966;96(4):546-50.

[43] Chang S, Yang S. Variability, related factors, and normal reference value of post-void residual urine in healthy kindergarteners. J Urol 2009;182:1933-8.

[44] Farhat W, Bägli DJ, Capolicchio G, O'Reilly S, Merguerian PA, Khoury A, McLorie GA. The dysfunctional voiding scoring system: Quantitative standardization of dysfunctional voiding symptoms in children. J Urol 2000;164(3 Pt 2):1011–5.

[45] Upadhyay J, Bolduc S, Bagli DJ, McLorie GA, Khoury AE, Farhat W. Use of the dysfunctional voiding symptom score to predict resolution of vesicoureteral reflux in children with voiding dysfunction. J Urol 2003;169(5):1842-46.

[46] Akbal C, Genc Y, Burgu B, Ozden E, Tekgul S. Dysfunctional voiding and incontinence scoring system: Quantitative evaluation of incontinence symptoms in pediatric population. J Urol 2005;173:969-73.

[47] Afshar K, Mirbagheri A, Scott H, MacNeily AE. Development of a symptom score for dysfunctional elimination syndrome. J Urol 2009;182(4 Suppl):939-43.

[48] Minardi D, Parri G, d'Anzeo G, Fabiani A, El Asmar Z, Muzzonigro G. Perineal ultrasound evaluation of dysfunctional voiding in women with recurrent urinary tract infections. J Urol 2008;179:947-51.

[49] de Jong TP, Klijn AJ, Vijverberg MA, de Kort LM, van Empelen R, Schoenmakers MA. Effect of biofeedback training on paradoxical pelvic floor movement in children with dysfunctional voiding. Urology. 2007;70(4):790-3.

[50] Chrzan R, Klijn AJ, Vijverberg MA, Sikkel F, de Jong TP. Colonic washout enemas for persistent constipation in children with recurrent urinary tract infections based on dysfunctional voiding. Urology 2008;71:607-10.

[51] Kibar Y, Demir E, Irkilata C, Ors O, Gok F, Dayanc M. Effect of biofeedback treatment on spinning top urethra in children with voiding dysfunction. Urology 2007;70(4):781-4.

[52] Sinha S. Dysfunctional voiding: A review of the terminology, presentation, evaluation and management in children and adults. Indian J Urol 2011;27(4):437-47.

[53] Wiener JS, Scales MT, Hampton J, King LR, Surwit R, Edwards CL. Long term efficacy of simple behavioral therapy for daytime wetting in children. J Urol 2000;164(3 Pt 1):786-90.

[54] Wennergren H, Oberg B, Sandstedt P. The importance of leg support for relaxation of the pelvic floor muscles: a surface electromyography study in healthy girls. Scand J Urol Nephrol 1991;25:205-13.

[55] Silva JM, Diniz JSS, Lima EM, Vergara RM, Oliveira EA. Predictive factors of resolution of primary vesico-ureteric reflux: a multivariate analysis. BJU Int 2006;97(5): 1063-8.

[56] Loening-Baucke V. Urinary incontinence and urinary tract infection and their resolution with treatment of chronic constipation of childhood. Pediatrics 1997;100(2 Pt 1): 228-32.

[57] Yagci S, Kibar Y, Akay O, Kilic S, Erdemir F, Gok F, Dayanc M. The effect of biofeedback treatment on voiding and urodynamic parameters in children with voiding dysfunction. J Urol 2005;174(5):1994-7.

[58] Desantis DJ, Leonard MP, Preston MA, Barrowman NJ, Guerra LA. Effectiveness of biofeedback for dysfunctional elimination syndrome in pediatrics: a systematic review. J Pediatr Urol 2011;7(3):342-8.

[59] Combs AJ, Glassberg AD, Gerdes D, Horowitz M. Biofeedback therapy for children with dysfunctional voiding. Urology 1998;52:312-5.

[60] Kibar Y, Piskin M, Irkilata HC, Aydur E, Gok F, Dayanc M. Management of abnormal postvoid residual urine in children with dysfunctional voiding. Urology 2010;75:1472-5.

[61] Curran MJ, Kaefer M, Peters C, Logigian E, Bauer SB. The overactive bladder in childhood: long-term results with conservative management. J Urol 2000;163:574-7.

[62] Willemsen J, Nijman RJ. Vesicoureteral reflux and videourodynamic studies: results of a prospective study. Urology 2000;55:939-43.

[63] Pohl HG, Bauer SB, Borer JG, Diamond DA, Kelly MD, Grant R, Briscoe CJ, Doonan G, Retik AB. The outcome of voiding dysfunction managed with clean intermittent

catheterization in neurologically and anatomically normal children. BJU Int 2002;89(9):923-7.

[64] Cain MP, Wu SD, Austin PF, Herndon CD, Rink RC. Alpha blocker therapy for children with dysfunctional voiding and urinary retention. J Urol 2003;170(4 Pt 2):1514-5.

[65] Kramer SA, Rathbun SR, Elkins D, Karnes RJ, Husmann DA. Double blind placebo controlled study of alpha-adrenergic receptor antagonists (doxazosin) for treatment of voiding dysfunction in the pediatric population. J Urol 2005;173(6):2121-4.

[66] Donohoe JM, Combs AJ, Glassberg KI. Primary bladder neck dysfunction in children and adolescents II: results of treatment with alpha-adrenergic antagonists. J Urol 2005;173(1):212-6.

[67] Schurch B, Hauri D, Rodic B, Curt A, Meyer M, Rossier AB. Botulinum-A toxin as a treatment of detrusor-sphincter dyssynergia: a prospective study in 24 spinal cord injury patients. J Urol 1996;155(3):1023-29.

[68] Mokhless I, Gaafar S, Fouda K, Shafik M, Assem A. Botulinum A toxin urethral sphincter injection in children with nonneurogenic neurogenic bladder. J Urol 2006;176(4 Pt 2): 1767-70.

[69] Steinhardt GF, Naseer S, Cruz OA. Botulinum toxin: Novel treatment for dramatic urethral dilatation associated with dysfunctional voiding. J Urol 1997;158(1):190-1.

[70] Franco I, Landau-Dyer L, Isom-Batz G, Collett T, Reda EF. The use of botulinum toxin A injection for the management of external sphincter dyssynergia in neurologically normal children. J Urol 2007;178(4 Pt 2):1775-9.

[71] Petronijevic V, Lazovic M, Vlajkovic M, Slavkovic A, Golubovic E, Miljkovic P. Botulinum toxin type A in combination with standard urotherapy for children with dysfunctional voiding. J Urol 2007;178(6):2599–602.

[72] Radojicic ZI, Perovic SV, Milic NM. Is it reasonable to treat refractory voiding dysfunction in children with botulinum-A toxin? J Urol 2006;176(1):332-6.

[73] Bower WF, Yeung CK. A review of non-invasive electro neuromodulation as an intervention or non-neurogenic bladder dysfunction in children. Neurourol Urodyn 2004;23:63-7.

[74] Roth TJ, Vandersteen DR, Hollatz P, Inman BA, Reinberg YE. Sacral neuromodulation for the dysfunctional elimination syndrome: A single center experience with 20 children. J Urol 2008;180:306-11.

[75] Humphreys MR, Vandersteen DR, Slezak JM, Hollatz P, Smith CA, Smith JE, Reinberg YE. Preliminary results of sacral neuromodulation in 23 children. J Urol 2006;176(5):2227-31.

[76] Killinger KA, Kangas JR, Wolfert C, Boura JA, Peters KM. Secondary changes in bowel function after successful treatment of voiding symptoms with neuromodulation. Neurourol Urodyn 2011;30:33-7.

[77] Capitanucci ML, Camanni D, Demelas F, Mosiello G, Zaccara A, De Gennaro M. Longterm efficacy of percutaneous tibial nerve stimulation for different types of lower urinary tract dysfunction in children. J Urol 2009;182(4 Suppl): 2056-61.

[78] Hagstroem S, Mahler B, Madsen B, Djurhuus JC, Rittig S. Transcutaneous electrical nerve stimulation for refractory daytime urinary urge incontinence. J Urol 2009;182(4 Suppl):2072-8.

Chapter 6

Functional Anatomy of the Vesicoureteric Junction: Implication on the Management of VUR/ UTI

Vivian Yee-Fong Leung and Winnie Chiu-Wing Chu

Additional information is available at the end of the chapter

http://dx.doi.org/10.5772/52168

1. Introduction

The detailed anatomy and the nature of the anti-reflux mechanism of the human vesicoureteric junction (VUJ) are still unknown and controversial. VUJ is traditionally thought to be a passive valve; however, recently there is increasing evidence to support the theory of a functional active neuro-muscular sphincter present at the VUJ. In this chapter, we sought to describe different forms of ureteric jet that can be visualized in both grey-scale and color Doppler ultrasound. We are going to summarize the results of a number of original studies based on large number of human subjects. From the observations of these studies, we propose the dual mode of action and an active functional sphincter at the VUJ.

2. Anatomy of Vesicoureteric Junction (VUJ)

The VUJ can be recognized as a small convex, bulging-out structure on the mucosal surface of the urinary bladder. The function of the VUJ is to allow unhindered antegrade passage of urine bolus from ureter into the bladder while prevent the reflux of urine into the ureter from the bladder, during both normal bladder filling and voiding.

2.1. Histology and histochemical study of the VUJ

The anatomical studies of human VUJ were first started around year 1800. To date, the mechanism of how VUJ functions is still poorly understood and controversies exist among different theories.

The generally accepted anatomical presentation of the VUJ is illustrated in a diagrammatic form as follows: (Fig 1).

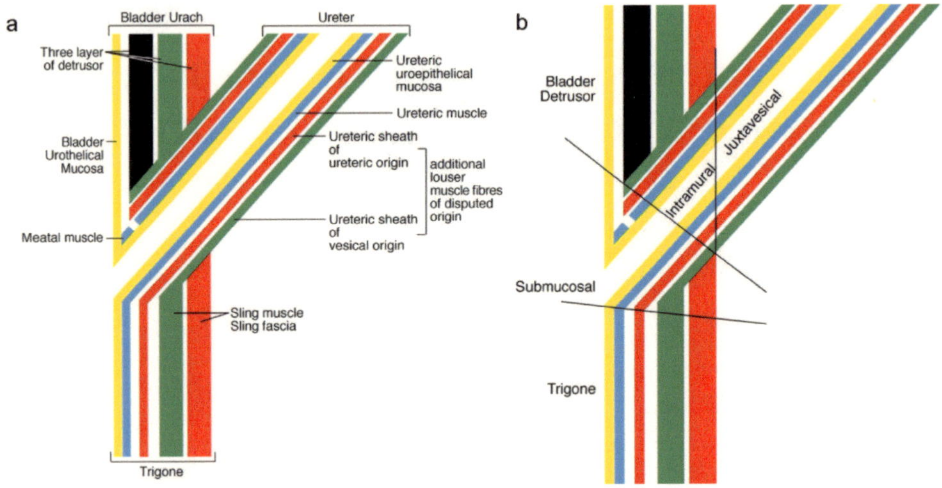

Figure 1. Schematic diagram of the anatomical layers in (a) ureteric and urinary bladder wall and (b) VUJ in human

2.1.1. Histology of the VUJ

VUJ involves three anatomical components: the ureteric wall, urinary bladder wall and the ureteric sheath. They are described as follows:

Three layers of ureteric and urinary bladder wall (Fig. 1a)

The wall of the ureter and urinary bladder consists of three layers: the outer adventitia, middle muscular layer and the inner mucosal layer.

The adventitia is the outermost layer composes of mainly fibrous connective tissues.

The muscular layer of the ureter consists of non-striated muscle which is uniform in thickness. When approaching the VUJ the muscle coat composes predominately longitudinally orientated muscle bundles (Gearhart et al., 1993). The ureteric muscle then fans out with fibers splitting around the orifice before becoming part of the superficial trigone. Some of the fibers extend to the urethra thereby creating connection between the urethra and the ureter (Bell's muscle) (Gearhart et al., 1993; Hutch et al., 1961; Juskiewenski et al., 1984; Noordzij & Dabhoiwala, 1993; Roshani et al., 1996; Stephens & Lenaghan, 1962; Tanagho & Pugh, 1963; Tanagho et al.,1968).

The muscular layer of the urinary bladder is also known as the detrusor muscle. It is composed of interlacing large bundles of non-striated muscle cell in a criss-cross arrangement. Different regions of the bladder have different muscle arrangements. There are anastomoses between different muscles in the form of complex reticular or netlike muscular meshwork. Four regions can be identified: the detrusor muscle proper, trigone, VUJ and the bladder neck.

The detrusor muscle proper consists of three ill-defined layers: an inner longitudinally orientated layer of muscle bundles, a substantial middle circular layer and an outer longitudinally orientated layer (Hunter, 1954; Uhlenhuth et al., 1953). The muscle fibers of the internal layer originate behind the ureteric orifice. The outer longitudinal bundles continue with the capsules of adjacent pelvic organs and the pubovesical ligament (Noordzij & Dabhoiwala, 1993). Three muscle layers of the detrusor form the superior part or roof of the VUJ. The inferior part or the floor is formed by only two layers of detrusor. They are the outer longitudinal layer (sling muscle) and the inner circular layer (sling fascia). They play an important role in the physiology of the VUJ by providing a firm support to the structures of the intravesical ureter and preventing reflux. They also form part of the trigone (Hutch et al., 1961; Tanagho & Pugh, 1963).

Finally the innermost mucosal layer of the ureter and the urinary bladder consists of a transitional epithelium (also known as the urothelium) and the lamina propria, the underlying supportive layer, consists of loose connective tissue. The urothelium is usually extensively folded, giving the ureteric lumen a satellite outline in histological specimens. However, this satellite pattern is not readily seen with ultrasound and may reflect a different process of collapse of the urothelium in vivo (Dyson, 1995; Motola et al., 1988; Tanagho, 2000).

Ureteric hiatus

The gap in the bladder wall through which the ureter passes is known as the ureteric hiatus. There are two gaps: outer and the inner hiatus. The outer hiatus is slightly higher and lateral to the inner hiatus. A roof and floor can also be identified. Thus the lower end of the ureter becomes oblique in position as it pierces through the bladder wall. The diagonal angle of passage of the ureter through the bladder wall in eight fresh human cadavers was 11^0 when using the endoluminal ultrasound method (Roshani et al., 1999). This cannot be confirmed in vivo because the angle of entry is only noticeable near the VUJ where the intramural channel is around 4-5 mm and more sharply angled than 11^0.

Different portion of the VUJ (Fig 1b)

There are two portions of ureter: The part outside the bladder muscle is known as the juxtavesical portion while inside is known as the intravesical portion. At birth, the intravesical ureter is 0.5 cm in length while in adulthood it is 1.5 to 2.6 cm. The intravesical ureter has two parts: the intramural and submucosal portion. The submucosal portion is covered by mucous membrane only. The intramural portion measures 0.9 cm while the submucosal part measures 0.7 cm in length. They are of approximately equal length in 80% at all ages (Cussen, 1967; Gruber, 1929; Hutch, 1961; Roshani et al., 1999; Tanagho & Pugh, 1963).

Ureteric Sheath (Fig. 1a)

There is an additional group of looser muscle fibers closely related to the adventitia of the intravesical and juxtavesical ureter, which is known as the ureteric sheath. This connective tissue sleeve separates the ureteric muscle coat from the bladder wall. However, the origin of this sheath is of great dispute. Some studies have suggested that the ureteric sheath is a separable structure. It is ureteric in origin and made by a fibromuscular layer wrapped around the intramural ureter (Disse, 1902; Tanagho & Pugh, 1963; Tanagho et al., 1968; Versari, 1908). Other studies have suggested that the sheath is vesical in origin, which is composed of longitudinal muscle fibers ascending from the bladder onto the juxtavesical part of the ureter (Hutch et al., 1961; Noordzij & Dabhoiwala, 1993; Uhlenhuth et al., 1953; Waldeyer, 1892).

Elbadawi and Ruotolo supported the dual sheath concept. They found two muscular sheaths surrounding the distal end of the ureter, superficial and deep periureteric sheaths. The superficial one was vesical in origin and the deep one was both ureteric and vesical in origin (Elbadawi, 1972; Ruotolo, 1949).

Other areas of the VUJ

There are also other areas about VUJ that are in dispute, including whether there is direct continuation of the trigone with ureter and the number of layers in trigonal muscle.

Some studies have suggested that the trigone is direct continuation with the ureter. The muscle fibers of the intravesical ureter fan out and become continuous with the superficial trigonal muscle. On the other hand, the ureteric sheath also fans out and joins the muscle bundles from the contralateral ureter forming the middle or deep trigone and extended to the urethra. This is called the Bell's muscle (Gruber, 1929; Juskiewenski et al., 1984; Noordzij & Dabhoiwala, 1993; Roshani et al., 1996; Tanagho & Pugh, 1963; Tanagho et al., 1968).

However, Disse, Uhlenhuth found that the ureteric muscle stopped abruptly in the VUJ thus they has proposed that the trigonal muscle is not of ureteric origin but represents submucous musculature (Disse, 1902; Uhlenhuth et al., 1953).

There is an isolated report on the existence of a sling muscle and meatal muscle in the VUJ (Fig 1a). Hutch has reported the existence of the sling muscle and sling fascia. They are the outer longitudinal and inner circular bladder muscles that form the floor of the VUJ and are thin but tough strip of muscle. These muscles lie underneath and provide firm support to the intravesical ureter, whichmight play a role in preventing reflux (Hutch et al., 1961).

Both Zaffagnini and Korner have reported the existence of the meatal muscle. There are transureteric vesical muscle bundles and extension of the deep periureteric sheath superficial to the ureteric muscle in the roof of the submucosal segment. The bundles of the two periureteric sheaths are cross or decussate with each other in the roof of the submucosal segment. This has been described as the meatal muscle (Zaffagnini & Mangiaracina, 1955) or a double perimeatal muscular sling (Korner, 1962).

Despite the controversies in different studies about the origin and relationships of the muscles, all studies do support the presence of muscle in the VUJ, thus suggesting that a potential functional muscular sphincter might be present.

2.1.2. Histochemical study of the VUJ

The VUJ has a dual sympathetic-parasympathetic innervation. It is richly supplied by noradrenergic and cholinergic nerves (Dixon et al., 1992, 1994, 1998a, 1998b; Gearhart et al., 1993; Gosling et al., 1999). The nerves supplying the ureterotrigonal and vesical component of the VUJ have the same origin: the ureterovesical ganglion complex. Therefore, theoretically the activity of the two components can be synchronized and regulated in relation to each other (Elbadawi & Schenk, 1971).

Both Jen and Roshani have shown that detrusor and deep trigone receive cholinergic innervation while the ureteric and superficial trigonal muscles receive noradrenergic innervation (Jen et al., 1995; Roshani et al., 1996) (Fig 2).

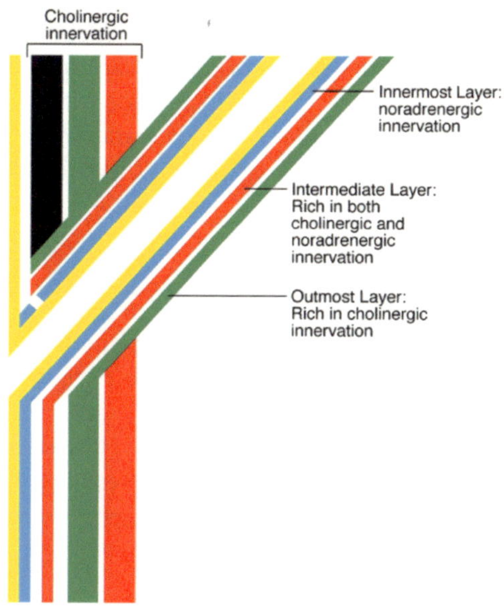

Figure 2. Histochemical study of the VUJ in human (according to Gearhart et al., 1993)

Gearhart have found three distinct smooth muscle components in the VUJ. The innermost layer is the ureteric muscle which is rich in pseudocholinesterase (PChE) and this muscle fans out and continues with the trigonal fiber. The intermediate layer of muscle is a distinct layer rich in both acetylcholinesterase (AChE) and PChE. It is not derived from the ureter or the detrusor but it continues with the trigonal fiber. The outermost layer is the detrusor muscle and is rich in AChE (Gearhart et al., 1993).

These additional informations further support our hypothesis that VUJ is likely to possess functional active sphincteric mechanism rather than just a passive flap valve.

2.2. Anti-reflux mechanism at VUJ

There are three well known schools of though for the anti-reflux mechanism: passive valve mechanism, mixed active and passive valvular action and sphincteric mechanism. However the exact nature of the anti-reflux mechanism of VUJ is unresolved and the existence of a valvular action is controversial.

2.2.1. *Passive valve mechanism*

Passive valve mechanism is a purely passive one which depends on the length and obliquity of the intravesicular ureter. When the intravesical pressure increases during bladder filling or voiding, there is an increase in length of the intravesical ureter and a one way "flap-valve" at the ureteric orifice is produced. The ureter is then compressed and flattened thus preventing regurgitation (Hutch, 1952; Hutch et al., 1955; Juskiewenski et al., 1984; Paquin, 1959).

2.2.2. Mixed active and passive valvular action

In this theory, the anti-reflux action depends on both the sphincter action of the bladder muscle and the obliquity of the ureter. The anti-reflux mechanism is brought by the dynamic relationship between bladder wall, intravesical ureter and trigone. (Blok et al., 1985, 1986; Hutch, 1952; Hutch et al., 1955, 1961; Roshani et al., 2000a, 2000b; Tanagho & Pugh, 1963; Tanagho et al.,1968).

2.2.3. Sphincteric mechanism

In this theory, the integrity of the VUJ is based on the sphincter action produced by the ureteric function and tone, and or urinary bladder action alone. The sphincteric action is brought by the muscular activity of the ureteric muscle, sling muscle, sling fascia and the Waldeyer's sheath and the intricate muscular meshwork of the trigonal region of the bladder (Hutch et al., 1961; Noordzij & Dabhoiwala, 1993; Stephens & Lenaghan, 1962; Stewart JC 1937; Tanagho & Pugh, 1963; Tanagho et al., 1968; Uhlenhuth et al., 1953).

3. Review of previous studies on ureteric jet

3.1. What is ureteric jet?

Ureteric jet is the forceful ejection of urine through the VUJ into the bladder and it can be detected by gray scale as a stream or burst of low-intensity echoes emerging from the ureteric orifice. The jet lasts for few seconds and it is fast enough to produce a frequency shift; thus both colour and Doppler waveform can be obtained at real-time (Fig 3)

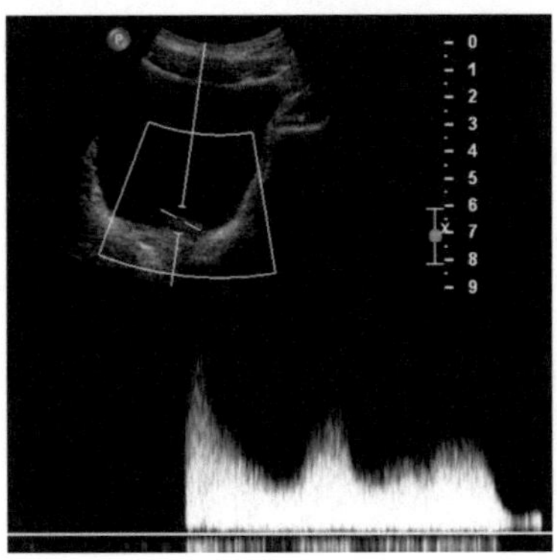

Figure 3. Colour and Doppler waveform of the ureteric jet.

http://dx.doi.org/10.5772/52168

Ureteric jet can be further characterized by its pulse wave Doppler waveform. In the next section, detailed literature review on ureteric jet in both human and animal studies will be outlined.

3.2. Previous work on the ureteric jet in human

Ureteric jet has been reported as early as 1955 (Kalmon et al., 1955) using the X-ray method (intravenous urography, IVU) while the first one to document the sonographic appearance of jet was Dubbins (Dubbins et al., 1981). The reported incidence of the visualization of jet ranged from 5.7% to 100% (Blomley et al., 1997; Cox et al., 1992; Eklöf & Johanson, 1980; Elejalde& de Elejalde, 1983; Gothlin, 1964; Marshall et al., 1990; Nevin et al., 1962). There is a higher chance of visualizing jet using ultrasound than radiography. Recently, the reported rate of visualization of ureteric jet in 1341 normal subjects using ultrasound is 99% (Leung et al., 2007b).

There are a number of theories why ureteric jet can be visualized on ultrasound, as follows: i) miniature bubbles produced in a rapidly moving fluid (Kremkau et al., 1970), ii) turbulent flow of urine into a static fluid in the closed bladder and the continual changes in the shear forces between the jet and the adjacent static urine was the caused for the Doppler signal (Dubbins et al., 1981), iii) difference in specific gravities of the injected fluid and the fluid within the bladder (Kremer et al., 1982), iv) differences in density and compressibility changes between urine in bladder and in the ureter (Baker & Middleton, 1992; Price et al., 1989).

3.2.1. Characteristics of ureteric jet

Pattern of the jet

There are many descriptions about Doppler waveform such as crescendo and decrescendo forms, single-hump and multiple-hump (as many as four) curves, turbulent form of jet pattern, discrete jets, ureteric streaming, rest periods (ie, period of undetected flow). Jet pattern could be divided into three phases: Firstly, initial phase can be visualized as pulsed oozing or flattened type or combination of both. It is then followed by a steady phase as uniform Doppler waveforms at regular intervals and a final phase as uneven waveforms at irregular intervals (Cox et al., 1992; Jequier et al., 1990; Wu et al., 1995). The pattern of jet alters with physiological changes. After large fluid load, there is eitheris an increase in jet frequency or the pattern is converted to an almost continuous signal with absent humps (Jequier et al., 1990). This temporal variation also occurs in velocity, duration and amplitude of the jet (Blomley et al., 1997; Burge et al., 1991; Cox et al., 1992; Wu et al., 1995).

On the contrary, during inadequate hydration or in diseased patients, the waveform becomes flattened (Wu et al., 1955).

Jets are usually directed anteriorly, anteromedially, with or without crossing of the jets. Sometimes they can also be perpendicular to the mucosal surface. There is not much difference in the jet direction bewteenboth paediatric and adult groups (Burge et al., 1991; Catalano et al., 1998; Cox et al., 1992; Dubbins et al., 1981; Elejalde & de Elejalde, 1983; Jequier et al., 1990; Patel & Kellett, 1996; Sweet et al., 1995).

Parameters of the jet

The extension of jet varies from 1 to 5 cm into the bladder but sometimes extended more than 5 cm or less than 1 cm (Dubbins et al., 1981; Elejalde & de Elejalde, 1983; Kremer et al., 1982).

The mean jet velocity in the paediatric group varies between 18 to 31.6 cm/s (from 26 days to 17 years old) while in the adults it varies from 32.1 to 60 cm/s (from 18 to 49 years old (Cox et al., 1992; Jequier et al., 1990; Marshall, 1990; Matsuda et al., 1995; Matsuda& Saitoh, 1995; Sperandeo et al., 1994;). The duration of jet ranges from 0.6 to 7.5 s (Jequier et al., 1990) in paediatric and from 3.5 to 15 s in adult (Catalano et al., 1998; Cox et al., 1992; Kremer et al., 1982; Matsuda et al., 1995). The frequency of jet ranges from 2.4 to 5.4 jets/min in adult (Burge et al., 1991; Catalano et al., 1998; Kremer et al., 1982; Matsuda & Saitoh, 1995). The interjet interval ranges from 2 to 150 seconds (Catalano et al., 1998; Cox et al., 1992).

Adult subjects have a higher velocity (20 vs. 16 cm/s), duration (2.5 vs. 1.8 s) and frequency (1.2 vs1 jets/min) than children (Matsuda & Saitoh., 1995).

There is symmetry in jet frequency, jet parameters of velocity and duration between right and left side in healthy subjects (Burge et al., 1991; Cox et al., 1992; Matsuda & Saitoh, 1995).

Under the condition of forced diuresis, the jet hasa higher velocity (32.1 vs. 20 cm/s), duration (6.7 vs. 2.5 s) and frequency (2.4 vs. 1.2 jets/min) than in the normal physiological state (Matsuda & Saitoh, 1995).

3.2.2. Clinical implication of ureteric jet

It has previously been suggested that the presence of ureteric jet implies concurrenturinary tract infection (UTI) (Kalmon et al., 1955; Nevin et al., 1962) and absence of vesicoureteric reflux (VUR) (Kuhns, 1977). Subsequent studies prove that the presence of ureteric jet is just a normal physiologic phenomenon and cannot be used to diagnosis UTI or exclude VUR (Eklöf & Johanson, 1980; Gothlin, 1964; Gudinchet et al., 1997; Jequier et al., 1990; Marshall et al., 1990).

However, the presence of jet could be used to exclude ureteric obstruction. The complete absence of jet or a continuous low-level waveform is diagnostic for high-grade obstruction from ureteric calculi (Abulafia et al., 1997; Burge et al., 1991; Catalano et al., 1998; Elejalde & de Elejalde, 1983; Laing et al., 1994; Tal et al., 1994; Timor-Tritsch et al., 1997; Wu et al., 1995; Yoon et al., 2000).The difference in jet velocity has been used to study the effect of drug treatment on benign prostatic hyperplasia (Sperandeo et al., 1994, 1996) and to study the physiology of the kidney and ureter, includingthe glomerular filtration rate (Blomley et al., 1997; Burke & Washowich, 1998; Chiu et al., 1999; Han et al., 1996, 1997; Patel et al., 1996; Summers et al., 1992; Wachsberg, 1998)

3.3. Previous work on the ureteric jet on animals

Lamb et al has found that ureteric jet can be consistently visualized in the dogs. The ureteric jets show variable frequency and duration. Lamb has suggested that the non-visualization of the ureteric jet might be helpful in diagnosing ectopic ureter (Lamb & Gregory, 1994).

http://dx.doi.org/10.5772/52168

In our institution, we have also studied the ureteric jet in 16s female pigs at the age of two to three monthsserially. The first scan was the baseline study, after that the pig underwent the process of deroofing of the intravesical portion on one of the ureters. The second scan was done one month after deroofing. The third scan was done when the pigs were four to five months old. The data from the pigs was compared with a group of 31 girls up to four years old. In this study, the incidence of monphasic waveform does not decrease as the pigs become mature. There is no association between reflux and monophasic waveform.

This observation is quite different from that in the human studies, as discussed in laterl part of this chapter.

4. Doppler waveform of ureteric jet

4.1. Pattern of the ureteric jet

Ureteric jets areclassified according to the number of peaks within that particular Doppler waveform. Six basic patterns are identified: monophasic (with only one peak), biphasic (two peaks), triphasic (three peaks), polyphasic (number of peaks exceeding three), "square" (a plateau waveform in which no distinct peak be identified but of average duration); and "continuous" when the waveform lasts longer than 20 seconds which can be either polyphasic or plateau form. These waveforms are further classified as three categories. Monophasic jet is classifies as the first category of simple and immature pattern (Fig. 4).

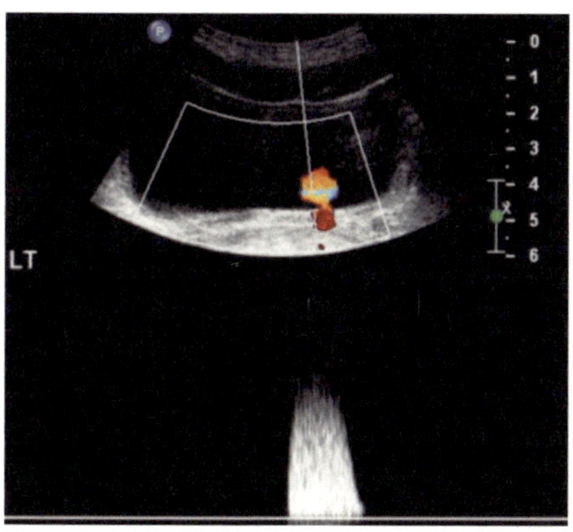

Figure 4. The simple, immature monophasic pattern of the ureteric jet

The bi, tri- and polyphasic patterns are classified as the complex and mature pattern (Fig 5).

The last two patterns are the square and continuous forms. These are modified waveform under the state of forced diuresis. They are classified as the diuretic pattern (Fig. 6).

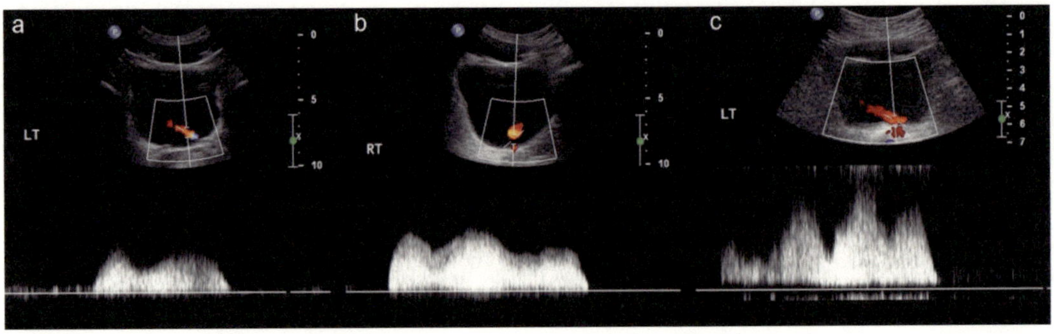

Figure 5. The complex and mature pattern of the ureteric jet: bi (a), tri (b), polyphasic (c)

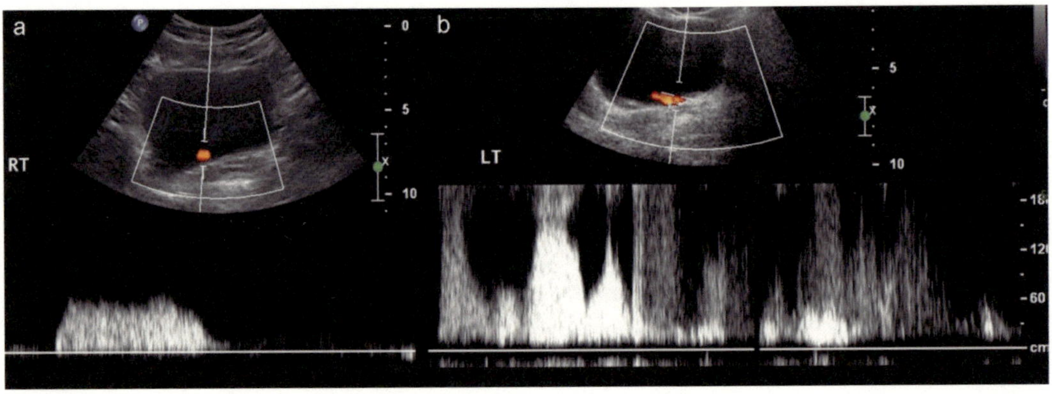

Figure 6. The diuretic pattern of the ureteric jet: square (a), continuous (b)

4.2. Measurement of ureteric jet

On the Doppler waveform, the maximum velocity (peak velocity), jet duration and initial slope can be measured (Fig 7).

4.3. Uncommon modification of the jet

There are three uncommon but interesting modifications of the jet. They are: presence of breaks, multispike pattern and change in direction of the jet. These patterns are relatively uncommon in the normal population but they provide indirect supportive evidence for the hypothesis of functional sphincter action at the VUJ.

Presence of breaks meant there is a total absence of signal between peaks within the duration of that particular wave (Fig 8). Most of the breaks are observed in the maximally full bladder and the incidence is found to be 5.7% of the study population (Leung et al., 2007b).

http://dx.doi.org/10.5772/52168

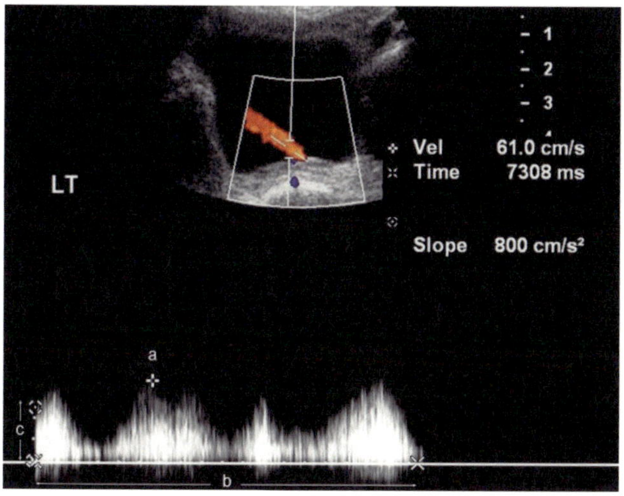

Figure 7. Doppler measurement of the ureteric jet: peak velocity (a), duration (b) and initial slope (c)

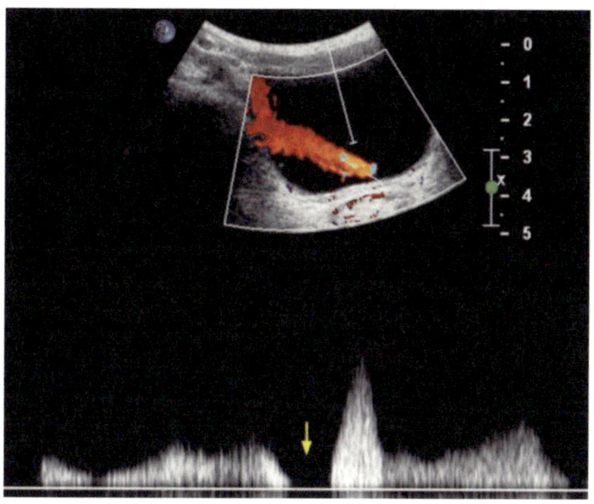

Figure 8. Presence of break (arrow) within the ureteric jet

Multispike pattern is defined as the pulsation in the jet pattern as a result of the pulsation transmitted from the adjacent arteries (Fig 9). This pattern is more commonly observed when bladder is maximally full and the incidence is found to be 1.9% of the study population (Leung et al., 2007b).

Change in angle of the jet meant there was a change in the direction of the jet at the beginning and at the end (Fig. 10). This pattern could be observed at any diuresis status. The incidence is found to be 4.3% of the study population (Leung et al., 2007b).

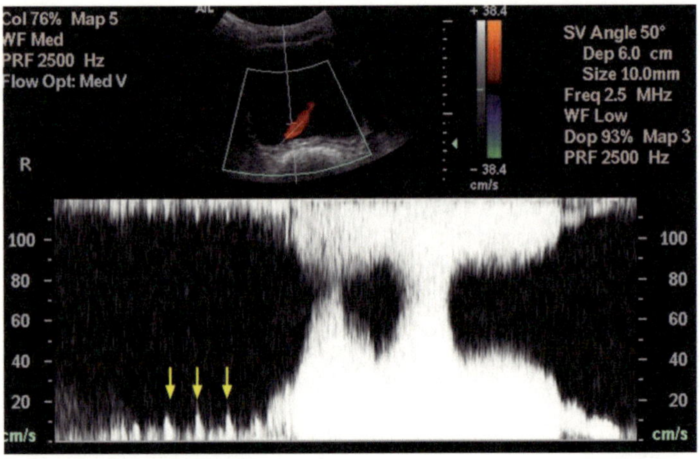

Figure 9. Multispike pattern (arrows) of the ureteric jet.

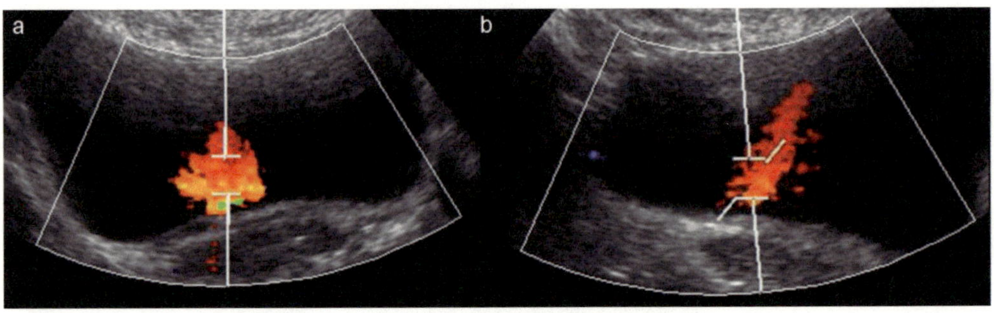

Figure 10. Changing of angle in the ureteric jet: from vertical at the beginning (a) to slightly inclined at the end (b) of the jet.

5. Our observation on Doppler waveform of the ureteric jet

In our institution, we have studied the pattern and physical properties of the ureteric jet in the normal population. The characteristics of ureteric jet are studied under specific physiological conditions such as pregnancy, pharmacological effect under general anaesthesia and after structural ureteric modification following renal transplantation. The characteristics of jet are also assessed under different pathological conditions such as: children with VUR and UTI, children with nocturnal enuresis and children with neurogenic bladder.

5.1. Physical properties of ureteric jet in normal population

This part of study is based on a normal population of 1,341 subjects with age ranging from 15 days to 82 years old (Leung et al., 2002a).

http://dx.doi.org/10.5772/52168

5.1.1. General properties of jet

In the normal population, four common patterns can be identified: monophasic, biphasic, triphasic and polyphasic (Table 1). The square and continuous patterns occur under force dieresis, which contributes only 1.5% of cases in the normal population. With increasing age from infancy, the proportion of monophasic waveform decreases while the more complex patterns prevail.

Age (year)	**Incidence (%)**			
	Monophasic	**Biphasic**	**Triphasic**	**Polyphasic**
0-9.9	30	30.6	23.3	16.1
10-19.9	3.3	28.7	41.1	26.9
20-29.9	0	35.6	40.7	23.7
30-39.9	2.0	35.6	35.1	27.3
40-49.9	2.5	34.1	32.7	30.7
50-59.9	3.8	38.7	30.8	26.7
60-69.9	0	38.0	35.5	26.4
70-79.9	4.7	37.2	37.2	20.9

Table 1. Incidence of the four patterns in different age groups of the normal population.

In the normal population, there is strikingly larger number of monophasic patterns in children (22%) than in adult (1.9%) (Table 2).

	Children		**Adult**	
	Number	**Incidence (%)**	**Number**	**Incidence (%)**
Monophasic	83	22	18	1.9
	P < 0.01			

Table 2. Incidence of monophasic jet in children and adult.

For the mean velocity, it is 34.03 cm/s for the monophasic jet and 61.82 cm/s for the complex pattern in children. While in adult, the mean velocity of the monophasic jet is 57.65 cm/s and 78.89 cm/s for the complex pattern.

For the mean jet duration, it is 1.17 s for children with monophasic pattern and 5.26 s for the complex pattern. In adults, the mean jet duration is 1.91 s for monophasic jet and 6.9 s for complex pattern.

For the mean initial slope, it is 211.82 cm/s^2 for monophasic jet and 293.32 cm/s^2 for the complex pattern in children. While in adults, the mean initial slope of the monophasic jet is 195.54 cm/s^2 and 271.21 cm/s^2 for the complex pattern.

The direction of flow of the jet can be directed anteriorly, anteromedially (with or without crossing of the jets), or in amore vertical direction or perpendicular to the bladder base.

5.1.2. Different effects on ureteric jet

The laterality differences, effect of age, gender and bladder filling status on the pattern of ureteric jet have been investigated.

In general, there is no significant difference in waveform pattern, initial slope, velocity and duration of ureteric jet between the right and left sides in both children and adults.

For the effect of age, children have a higher incidence of monophasic jet. This immature pattern occurs constantly in the first 6 months of life and becomes mature at the age of 4.54 years. There is no significant gender difference for the mean age of VUJ maturity in children (Leung et al., 2007a). Adults have higher jet velocity and longer duration of jet than children for both the monophasic and complex patterns. However, the initial slope of the jet shows no significant difference between children and adults.

For the gender effect, in children, there is no significant difference in velocity, duration, initial slope or number of peaks within a single jet between boys and girls. In adults, male subjects have a higher incidence of polyphasic waveform than females involving both right and left side. Male subjects also have a higher velocity and longer duration of the jet than female on both sides.

Finally, as for the effect of bladder filling status on the jet, 42.2% of subjects show no change in the number of peaks within a single jet waveform, 28.9% show a decrease and 26.5% show an increase, and 2.4% has square and continuous jet when the bladder becomes very full (Leung et al., 2002a). In all subjects, the initial slope, velocity and duration of the jet are not affected by different stages of bladder filling. In conclusion, the stage of bladder filling should have little effect to determine whether a subject has an immature or complex pattern.

5.2. Characteristic of the jet in different physiological conditions

5.2.1. Physiological effect

Hormonal changes of pregnancy are thought to cause smooth muscle relaxation (Hundley et al., 1942; Kumar, 1962). In our institution, we sought to investigate whether this hormonal effect on the smooth muscle exists within the maternal urinary tract, if the hypothesis of a functional active sphincteric mechanism at the VUJ is sound. A longitudinal study has been used to illustrate this physiological change. A total of 107 pregnant women have performed Doppler study of the ureteric jet at 20, 32 weeks' gestation, and 3 months postpartum. The incidence of monophasic jet (immature jet) is significantly higher at 20 weeks' gestation (18.7%), and even higher at 32 weeks' gestation (41.1%) when compared with non-pregnant women (1.9%). However, the incidence drops to again and becomes comparable to the non-pregnant women (1.6% vs. 1.9%) after 3-month postpartum (Leung & Metreweli, 2002a).

In the above study, we conclude that pregnancy does modify the ureteric jet pattern. One possible explanation is that the VUJ reverts to the simpler mechanism to produce the monophasic pattern by the myogenic component when the mature neural component fails or is inactivated to produce complex jet pattern. Therefore the complex ureteric jet is subject to an on-off switch. If it is switched off then the ureter reverts back to a monophasic jet. The above observation leads to the hypothesis about a myogenic origin related to the monophasic waveform and a neurogenic origin related to the complex waveform.

5.2.2. Pharmacological effect

Another study has been set to investigate for any effect of the anaesthesia drug on functional sphincteric action of the VUJ. If so, this will be reflected by changes in the Doppler waveform of the ureteric jet after application of anaesthesia. We have studied a total of 16 children while they underwent surgery under general anaesthesia. Before anaesthesia, 14 of them showed a complex pattern and two showed a monophasic pattern. However, after anaesthesia, all of them showed a monophasic waveform (Leung et al., 2003).

This observation confirms that the change in the ureteric jet from a complex to a monophasic waveform is brought by the effect of the drugs acting on the functional sphincteric action of the VUJ. This observation again supports the hypothesis of a functional active sphincter and supports the dual components of the VUJ sphincter. In this scenario, the neural component of the VUJ is inactivated by the anaesthesia, leaving only the myogenic component to function, hence producing the monophasic jet pattern.

5.2.3. Structural modification effect

Ureteric peristalsis in the transplanted ureter should be the same as that in the normal subject. The traditional concept about VUJ competence is mechanical in origin, so that during re-implantation of the donor ureter into the native bladder, the structure or function of the native VUJ is destroyed and the equivalent of a mechanical flap valve is "re-created" (Paquin, 1959; Politano et al., 1958). However, no one has studied whether the surgical VUJ behaves in a similar manner as a native VUJ. In our institution, we have assessed for any change in the ureteric jet after ureteric transplantation for renal transplantation, so as to demonstrate the effect of structural change at VUJ.

The ureteric jets from 55 renal transplant patients have been compared with 817 healthy subjects. The Doppler waveform of transplant ureters is distinctly different from those of healthy adult ureters. Only two patterns can be identified in transplanted ureters: more commonly a short monophasic waveform (66.1% vs. 2.6% in the health ureters), and less commonly a longer multiphase pattern but does not resemble the patterns of the healthy ureter (Leung & Metreweli, 2002b).

In conclusion, the ureteric jet patterns associated with transplant ureters are very different from those ureters with an intact VUJ, but resemble the pattern expected from simple efflux of urine secondary to ureteric peristalsis. On the other hand, this jet pattern of transplanted ureter also has little resemblance to the normal monophasic pattern because the latter requires some functional sphincteric type activity, referred as myogenic component in the dual component theory that we have described earlier. Furthermore the more complicated transplant jet bears no resemblance to the normal complex category. This can be explained by the loss of the proposed neural component. Inherent ureteric muscular peristalsis has been shown to be preserved in transplanted ureter, which is likely to be the vis-a-tergo producing the jet. In conclusion, there is a loss of functional active sphincter mechanism of the VUJ in the transplanted ureter as a result of the operative procedure. This observation again supports the hypothesis that VUJ is a functional active sphincter.

5.3. Characteristic of the ureteric jet in different pathological condition

Characteristic of Doppler waveform of the ureteric jet in different pathological groups have also been investigated, as illustrated below.

5.3.1. Children with VUR and UTI

We have previously shown that young children have a much simpler monophasic immature pattern. A study has been carried out to study whether there is any correlation between the presence of such immature pattern with UTI and VUR.

We have studied 98 children with UTI and VUR and compared with 241 healthy children. The incidence of monophasic jet (immature pattern) is 29% in healthy children overall, but varies greatly according to age. The immature pattern is universal in the first 6 months of life, but drops significantly to below 15% in late childhood. This immature pattern is more commonly seen in children with UTI (37.5%) and VUR (90.5%) than in healthy controls of the same age (Leung et al., 2002b).

An immature pattern of ureteric jet is seen predominantly in three groups of subjects: (1) neonatal and infant group, (2) children with UTI and (3) children with VUR,. However in older children between 2-14 years of age, there is a higher tendency of persist immature pattern in both UTI and VUR groups. The persistence of immature jet pattern suggests that developmental immaturity might be a feature of children with UTI and VUR.

As immature ureteric jet pattern is associated with immaturity of ureteric function during infancy, a similar pattern observed in UTI / VUR groups lead to a hypothesis that this developmental immaturity of VUJ might be a contributing/ predisposing factor to urinary infection and the reflux problem in children.

Previous studies have been that majority of children with VUR do not have an anatomically defined congenital anomaly at the VUJ, (Dixon et al., 1998a), however, a functionally immature or transitory phase of developmental immaturity of VUJ might be present and predispose the affected children to VUR and UTI.

http://dx.doi.org/10.5772/52168

5.3.2. *Children with nocturnal enuresis*

In our institution, a study has been set to investigate whether immature ureteric jet pattern is present in children with nocturnal enuresis.

We have studied 511 children presenting with primary nocturnal enuresis. There was a higher incidence (19%) of immature waveform observed in children with nocturnal enuresis as compared with normal children within the same age range (7.4%) (Leung et al 2006). This study suggests that there is a lower level of maturity in the VUJ in enuretic children. Another interesting finding is that the immature jet is more commonly seen in enuretic children with markedly thickened bladder wall and multiple urodynamic abnormalities. This observation suggests that monophasic waveform is associated with abnormalities of the detrusor muscle as well as an increase in detrusor pressure. All these parameters might be indicators of immaturity of the VUJ-detrusor complex, which predispose affected children to the development of primary enuresis.

5.3.3. *Children with neurogenic bladder*

As discussed previously, VUJ has a nervous component with hitherto unknown functions. Patients with inactivated neural component within the VUJ due to drug effects or surgery have a higher incidence of monophasic jet pattern. It is well known that patients with neurogenic bladder have high incidence of secondary VUR while VUR is associated with monophasic ureteric jet. In our institution, we sought to investigate whether there is a prevalence of monophasic jet in patients with neurogenic bladder.

In a study of 27 children with neurogenic bladder, the frequency of monphasic jet is much higher in neurogenic bladder group (40.7%) when compared with normal population within the same age range (7%). Despite the small number of subjects, the observation again supports the theory of functional active sphincteric mechanism of VUJ. In this scenario, monophasic pattern prevails when the neural component within the VUJ is deactivated.

6. Dual mode of action of the functional sphincter at the VUJ

In summary, combining the anatomical and histochemical data, as well as the observations from Doppler ultrasound studies of ureteric jets, a functional sphincter with dual mode action at the VUJ is proposed. This sphincter is not a passive valve. On top of the monophasic ureteric peristaltic wave within the ureters as demonstrated by M-mode, a more complex pattern is observed in the ureteric jet emanating from VUJ demonstrated by Doppler waveform. The reason for the change in waveform pattern of the ultimate ureteric jet is due to modification of jet by an active sphincter mechanism at the VUJ.

In brief, six patterns of ureteric jet and three uncommon variations are identified. They are classified as the monophasic, mature complex (bi, tri and polyphasic) and diuretic pattern. In the normal population, a higher incidence of the monophasic pattern is seen in immature neonate and in children under four years old. The monophasic pattern occurs constantly in the first six months of life. There is a significant drop in the incidence of monophasic pattern by the age of four. The complex waveforms prevail in older children and normal adults. There are two components in the dual mode action of such functional sphincter. They are the "myogenic" (primary or immature) component and the "neurogenic" (secondary or mature) component. We postulate that the monophasic jet pattern is the result of contraction caused by the myogenic component of the VUJ, while the complex pattern is the result of modulation of the myogenic component of the jet by the neurogenic component in response to the distal intrauretetic pressure (Fig 11). The mode of the functional sphincteric action of the VUJ and the subsequent ureteric jet waveform vary depending upon whether or not the neurogenic component is active.

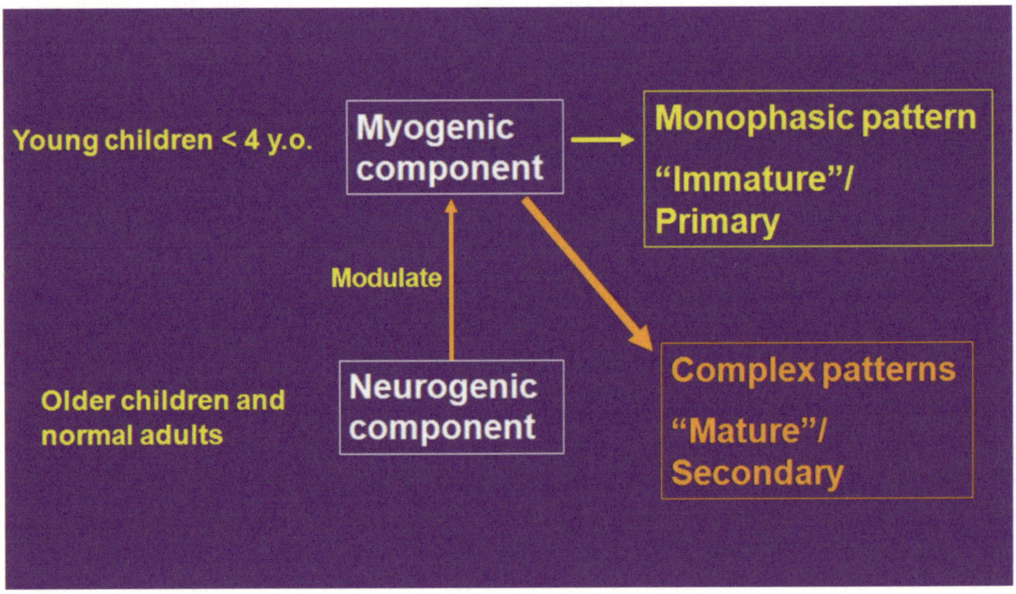

Figure 11. Diagram showing the dual mode of action of the VUJ in the normal population

The presence of the less frequently observed modifications of the ureteric jet pattern is also contributed to the dual mode action of VUJ. The multispike pattern appears to be a premature relaxation of the VUJ that precedes the ureteric jet proper. It is related to the relaxation mechanism found in forced diuresis. Forced diuresis is probably caused by permanent relaxation of the VUJ functional sphincter allowing free flow of urine modified by ureteric peristalsis. These modifications are under the control of neural mechanism. The breaks modification is found under condition of maximum bladder filling hence increased intravesical pressure. This is probably a result of the pressure wave of the ureteric jet generating apparently lower velocities and intervening with zero flows.

Whenever the neurogenic component is switched off, only the myogenic component operates and thus results in a reversion to the monophasic pattern of the ureteric jet. The above holds true under three physiological conditions. During pregnancy, the hormonal

http://dx.doi.org/10.5772/52168

effect temporarily inactivates the neurogenic component. Once the hormonal effect is lost, the neural component is activated again. In the anaesthetized (GA) children, the drug effect also temporarily inactivated the neurogenic component. In patients undergoing renal transplantation, the normal VUJ mechanism in the transplant ureter is altered or completely lost as a result of the operative procedure, thus a totally different ureteric jet pattern is observed (Fig 12).

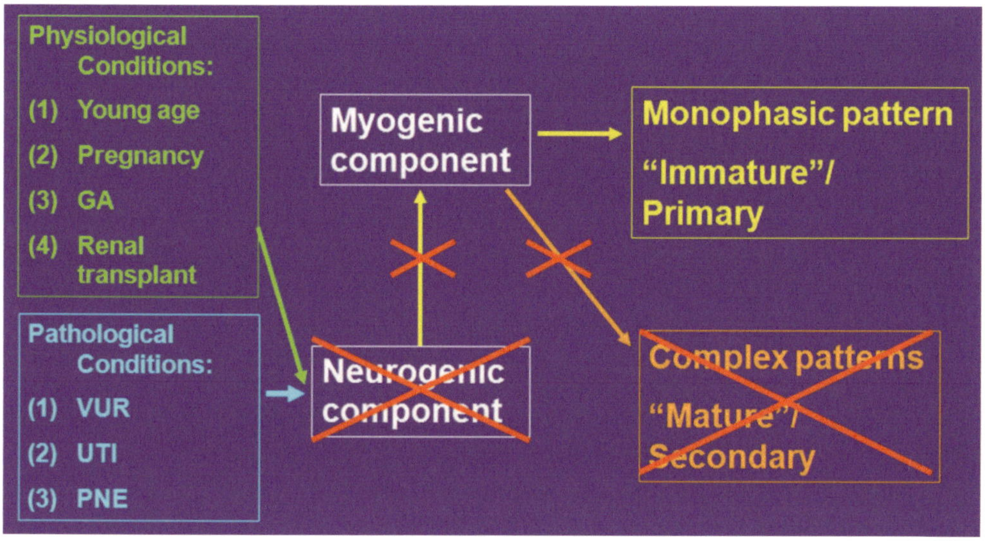

Figure 12. Diagram showing the inactivation of the neurogenic component under different physiological and pathological conditions

Under pathological conditions, there is strong correlation between the presence of VUR and the immature monophasic waveform. This suggests that the more mature complex jet pattern is associated with a more efficient anti-reflux mechanism than the simple immature pattern. The immature jet pattern may represent a temporary developmental immaturity of the VUJ, which predisposes children to the risk of VUR. Monophasic jet is also found in children with nocturnal enuresis associated with detrusor immaturity. A higher incidence of monophasic waveform is also found in children with neurogenic bladder, consistent with loss of the neural component. This might also explain why there is a higher incidence of VUR and UTI in children with neurogenic bladder when the anti-reflux mechanism is lost at the VUJ (Fig 12).

7. Conclusion

The concept of dual mode action (myogenic and neurogenic component) of a functional active sphincter at human VUJ has the following implications:

1. Human VUJ function takes time to mature.

2. It is important for understanding the physiology of VUJ and the mechanism for predisposition to certain pathological conditions, such as VUR and UTI in children

3. This may change the traditional thinking and management of VUR and UTI in children and adults. For example, as the normal physiology of the functional sphincter action of the VUJ is affected by anaesthesia, any VUR study performed in an anaesthetized child should be abandoned (The situation in adults is not known).

4. It is a potentially useful clinical tool for identifying children who are at risk of developing VUR and UTI. This mightlead to more aggressive intervention that will protect the upper urinary tract before any damage is sustained.

5. It is a potentially useful non-invasive investigation to assess bladder abnormalities in children with nocturnal enuresis. It may also enable evaluation of the efficiency of pharmacological interventions.

6. As the VUJ functional sphincter share components of the detrusor muscle, study of ureteric jet may also reflect detrusor activity and the effects of pharmacological intervention on the detrusor.

As a conclusion, the implication of this chapter is that it will alter the scientific basis in the understanding of VUJ and related pathological conditions.. Doppler ultrasound study of ureteric jet provides a non-invasive, physiological and ethical method to study the physiology and pathophysiology of VUJ. In the future, this is valuable for evaluating the therapeutic approach in different kinds of pathological conditions related to VUJ and bladder detrusor activity.

Author details

Vivian Yee-Fong Leung and Winnie Chiu-Wing Chu

The Chinese University of Hong Kong, Prince of Wales Hospital, Hong Kong, SAR

References

[1] Abulafia, O., Sherer, D. M., & Lee, P. S. (1997). Postoperative Color Doppler Flow Ultrasonographic Assessment of Ureteral Patency in Gynecologic Oncology Patients. *J Ultrasound Med.16*, 125-9.

[2] Baker, S. M., & Middleton, W. D. (1992). Color Doppler Sonography of Ureteral Jets in Normal Volunteers: Importance of the Relative Specific Gravity of Urine in the Ureter and Bladder. AJR., 159, 773-5.

[3] Blok, C., Van Venrooij, G. E. P. M., & Coolsaet, B. L. R. A. (1985). Dynamics of the ureterovesical junction; effectiveness of its ureteral peristalsis in high pressure pig bladders. J Urol., 134, 825-7.

[4] Blok, C., Van Venrooij, G. E. P. M., Mokhless, I., & Coolsaet, B. L. R. A. (1986). Dynamics of the ureterovesical junction:its resistance to upper urinary tract outflow in pigs. J Urol. , 136, 1127-31.

[5] Blomley, M. J. K., Ramsey, C. M., Cosgrove, , Patel, N., Lynch, M., Glass, D. M., & Peters, A. M. (1997). The Ureteric Jet Index: a Novel measure of Divided Renal Function. Clin Radiol. , 52, 771-4.

[6] Burge, H. J., Middleton, W. D., Mc Clennan, B. L., & Hildebolt, C. F. (1991). Ureteral Jets in Healthy Subjects and in Patients with Unilateral Ureteral Calculi: Comparison with Color Doppler US. Radiology., 180, 437-42.

[7] Burke, B. J., & Washowich, T. L. (1998). Ureteral Jets in Normal Second-and Third-Trimester Pregnancy. J Clin Ultrasound , 26, 423-6.

[8] Catalano, O., De Sena, G., & Nunziata, A. (1998). The color Doppler US evaluation of the ureteral jet in patients with urinary colic. Radiol Med (Torino)., 95, 614-7.

[9] Chiu, N. T., Wu, C. C., Yao, W. J., Tu, D. G., Lee, B. F., Tong, Y. C., & Pan, C. C. (1999). Evaluation and Validation of Ureteric Jet Index by Glomerular Filtration Rate. Invest Radio. , 34, 499-502.

[10] Cox, I. H., Erickson, S. J., Foley, W. D., & Dewire, D. M. (1992). Ureteric Jets: Evaluation of Normal Flow Dynamics with Color Doppler Sonography. AJR., 158, 1051-5.

[11] Cussen, L. J. (1967). Dimensions of the normal ureter in infancy and childhood. J Urol. , 5, 164-78.

[12] Diess, J. (1902). Nierenbecken und Harnleiter. In Handbuch der Anatomie des Menschen. Jene: Gustav Fishcer.Band VIII/I:, 105-112.

[13] Dixon, J. S., Canning, D. A., Gearhart, J. P., & Goslilng, J. A. (1994). An immuno- histochemical study of the innervation of the ureterovesical junction in infancy and childhood. Br J Urol. , 73, 292-7.

[14] Dixon, J. S., Goslilng, J. A., Canning, D. A., & Gearhart, J. P. (1992). An immuno- histochemical study of human postnatal paraganglia associated with the urinary bladder. J Anat. , 181, 431-6.

[15] Dixon, J. S., Jen, P. Y. P., & Goslilng, J. A. (1998a). Immunohistochemical characteristics of human paraganglion cells and sensory corpuscles associated with the urinary bladder. A developmental study in the male fetus, neonate and infant. J Anat., 192, 407-15.

[16] Dixon, J. S., Jen, P. Y. P., Yeung, C. K., Chow, L. T. C., Mathwes, R., Gearhart, J. P., & Goslilng, J. A. (1998b). The structure and autonomic innervation of the vesico-ureteric junction in cases of primary ureteric reflux. Br J Urol., 81, 146-51.

[17] Dubbins, P. A., Kurtz, A. B., Darby, J., & Goldberg, B. B. (1981). Ureteric Jet Effect: The Echogenic Appearance of Urine Entering the Bladder. Radiology., 140, 513-5.

[18] Dyson, M. (1995). Ch 13 Urinary System. In Williams PL et al ed Gray's anatomy. 38th Ed. Churchill Livingstone.

[19] Eklöf, O. A., & Johanson, L. (1980). Occurrence of Reflux in Children with Ureteral Jets. Pediatr Radiol., 10, 95-9.

[20] Elbadawi, A. (1972). Anatomy and function of the ureteral sheath. J Urol., 102, 224-9.

[21] Elbadawi, A., & Schenk, E. A. (1971). A new theory of the innervation of bladder musculature. Part 2. The innervation apparatus of the ureterovesical junction. J Urol., 105, 368-71.

[22] Elejalde, B. R., & de Elejalde, . (1983). Ureteral Ejaculation of Urine Visualized by Ultrasound. J Clin Ultrasound., 11, 475-6.

[23] Gearhart, J. P., Canning, D. A., Gilpin, S. A., Lam, , & Goslilng, J. A. (1993). Histological and Histochemical Study of the Vesicoureteric Junction in Infancy and Childhood. Br J Urol., 72, 648-54.

[24] Goslilng, J. A., Dixon, J. S., & Jen, P. Y. P. (1999). The distribution of Noradrenergic Nerves in the Human Lower Urinary Tract. Eur Urol., 36, 23-30.

[25] Gothlin, J. (1964). Ureteral Jets. Radiologe., 4, 398-400.

[26] Gruber, C. M. (1929). I. A comparative study of the intra-vesical ureters (uretero-vesical valves) in man and in experimental animals. J Urol., 21, 567-81.

[27] Gudinchet, F., Oberson, J. C., & Frey, P. (1997). Color Doppler Ultrasound for Evaluation of Collagen Implants after Endoscopic Injection Treatment of Refluxing Ureters in Children. J Clin Ultrasound., 25, 201-6.

[28] Han, S. J., Wu, C. C., Tsai, C. C., Yao, W. J., & Wang, S. C. (1997). Ureteral Jet Index in the Assessment of Renal Function. J Med Ultrasound., 5, 45-8.

[29] Han, S. J., Wu, C. C., Yao, W. J., Mo, L. R., Tsai, C. C., & Hwang, M. H. (1996). Ureteral Jet Index in 50 Normal Subjects and 11 Patients with Renoureteral Abnormalities. J Med Ultrasound., 4, 124-8.

[30] Hundley, J. M., Diehl, W. K., & Diggs, E. S. (1942). Hormonal influences upon the ureter. Am J Obstet Gynecol., 44, 858-72.

[31] Hunter De, W. T. (1954). A new concept of urinary bladder musculature. J Urol. , 71, 695-704.

[32] Hutch, J. A. (1952). Vesico-ureteral reflux in the paraplegic: cause and correction. J Urol., 68, 457-69.

[33] Hutch, J. A. (1961). Theory of maturation of the intravesical ureter. J Urol. , 86, 534-8.

[34] Hutch, J. A., Bunge, R. G., & Flocks, R. H. (1955). Vesicoureteral reflux in children. J Urol. , 74, 607-20.

[35] Jen, P. Y. P., Dixon, J. S., & Goslilng, J. A. (1995). Immunohistochemical localization of neuromarkers and neuropeptides in human fetal and neonatal urinary bladder. Br J Urol. , 75, 230-5.

[36] Jequier, S., Paltiel, H., & Lafortune, M. (1990). Ureterovesical Jets in Infants and Children: Duplex and Color Doppler US studies. Radiology., 175, 349-53.

[37] Juskiewenski, S., Vaysse, P., Moscovici, J., de Graeve, P., & Guitard, J. (1984). The ureterovesical junction. Anatomia Clinica., 5, 251-9.

[38] Kalmon, E. H., Albers, D. D., & Dunn, J. H. (1955). Ureteral Jet Phenomenon. Stream of Opaque Medium Simulating an Anomalous Configuration of the Ureter. Radiology. , 65, 933-5.

[39] Korner, F. (1962). Zur funktionellen Struktur des Ureters unter besonderer Beruchsichtigung seines distalen Endes. Verhandl Anat Gesellsch.58:169.

[40] Kremer, H., Dobrinski, W., Mikyska, M., Baumgartner, M., & Zollner, N. (1982). Ultrasonic in Vivo and in Vitro Studies on the Nature of the Ureteral Jet Phenomenon. Radiology., 142, 175-7.

[41] Kremkau, F. W., Gramiak, R., Carstensen, E. L., Shah, P. M., & Kramer, D. H. (1970). Ultrasonic Detection of Cavitation at Catheter Tips. Am J Radiology., 110, 177-83.

[42] Kuhns, L. R., Hernandez, R., Koff, S., Thornbury, J. R., Poznanski, A. K., & Holt, J. F. (1977). Absence of Vesico-Ureteral Reflux in Children with Ureteral Jets. Radiology., 124, 185-7.

[43] Kumar, D. (1962). In vitro inhibitory effect of progesterone on extrauterine human smooth muscle. Am J Obstet Gynecol., 84, 1300-4.

[44] Laing, F. C., Benson, C. B., Di Salvo, D. N., Brown, D. L., Frates, M. C., & Loughlin, K. R. (1994). Distal Ureteral Calculi: Detection with Vaginal US. Radiology., 192, 545-8.

[45] Lamb, C. R., & Gregory, S. P. (1994). Ultrasonography of the ureterovesical junction in the dog: a preliminary report. Vet Rec., 134, 36-38.

[46] Leung, V. Y. F., & Metreweli, C. (2002a). Doppler waveform of the ureteric jet in pregnancy. Ultrasound Med Biol. , 28, 879-84.

[47] Leung, V. Y. F., & Metreweli, C. (2002b). Ureteric jet in renal transplantation patient. Ultrasound Med Biol. , 28, 885-8.

[48] Leung, V. Y. F., Metreweli, C., & Yeung, C. K. (2002a). The ureteric jet Doppler waveform as an indicator of vesicoureteric sphincter function in adults and children. An observational study. Ultrasound Med Biol. , 28, 865-72.

[49] Leung, V. Y. F., Metreweli, C., & Yeung, C. K. (2002b). Immature ureteric jet Doppler patterns and urinary tract infection and vesico-ureteric reflux in children. Ultrasound Med Biol. , 28, 873-8.

[50] Leung, V. Y. F., Metreweli, C., Yeung, C. K., & Sihoe, J. D. Y. (2003). Ureteric jet in the anaesthetised child. Ultrasound Med Biol. , 29, 1237-1240.

[51] Leung, V. Y. F., Chu, W. C. W., Yeung, C. K., & Metreweli, C. (2006). Ureteric jet Doppler Waveform and Bladder Wall Thickness in Children with Nocturnal Enuresis. Pediatr Res , 60, 582-586.

[52] Leung, V. Y. F., Chu, W. C. W., Yeung, C. K., & Metreweli, C. (2007a). Gender difference in achieving rate of maturity of the vesicoureteric junction. Pediatr Radiol , 37, 189-193.

[53] Leung, V. Y. F., Chu, W. C. W., Yeung, C. K., & Metreweli, C. (2007b). Doppler waveforms of the ureteric jet: an overview and implications for the presence of a functional sphincter at the vesicoureteric junction. Pediatr Radiol , 37, 417-425.

[54] Marshall, J. L., Johnson, N. D., & De Campo, M. P. (1990). Vesicoureteric Reflux in Children: Prediction with Color Doppler Imaging. Work in Progress. Radiology., 175, 355-8.

[55] Matsuda, T., & Saitoh, M. (1995). Detection of the Urine Jet Phenomenon Using Doppler Color Flow Mapping. Int J Urol., 2, 232-4.

[56] Motola, J. A., Shahon, R. S., & Smith, A. D. (1988). Anatomy of the Ureter. Urol Clin North Am., 15, 295-9.

[57] Nevin, I. N., Cline, F. A., & Haug, T. M. (1962). Forceful Ureteral Spurt. A Common Roentgen Manifestation of Urinary Tract Infection in Children. Radiology. , 79, 933-8.

[58] Noordzij, J. W., & Dabhoiwala, N. F. (1993). A view of the anatomy of the ureterovesical junction. Scand J Urol Nephrol., 27, 371-80.

[59] Paquin, A. J. (1959). Ureterovesical anastomosis: The description and evaluation of a technique. J Urol., 82, 573-83.

[60] Patel, U., & Kellett, . (1996). Ureteric drainage and peristalsis after stenting studied using color Doppler ultrasound. Br J Urol., 77, 530-5.

[61] Price, C. I., Adler, R. S., & Rubin, J. M. (1989). Ultrasound Detection of Difference in Density Explanation of the Ureteric Jet Phenomenon and Implications for New Ultrasound Applications. Invest Radiol., 24, 876-83.

[62] Roshani, H., Dabhoiwala, N. F., Dijkhuis, T., Kurth, K. H., & Lamers, W. H. (2000a). An in vivo endoluminal ultrasonographic study of peristaltic activity in the distal porcine ureter. J Urol.163:602.

[63] Roshani, H., Dabhoiwala, N. F., Dijkhuis, T., Ongerboer de, Visser. B. W., Kurth, K. H., & Lamers, W. H. (2000b). An electro-myographic study of the distal porcine ureter. J Urol., 163, 1570-6.

[64] Roshani, H., Dabhoiwala, N. F., Verbeek, F. J., Kurth, K. H., & Lamers, W. H. (1999). Anatomy of ureterovesical junction and distal ureter studied by endoluminal ultrasonography in vitro. J Urol., 161, 1614-9.

[65] Roshani, H., Dabhoiwala, N. F., Verbeek, F. J., & Lamers, W. H. (1996). Functional Anatomy of the Human Ureterovesical Junction. The Anat Rec., 245, 645-51.

[66] Ruotolo, A. (1949). Sul signiticato morfologico e funzionale della guaina ureterale e della considetta fessure del valdeyer. Urologia., 16, 9-17.

[67] Sperandeo, M.., Varriale, A., Sperandeo, G., Caturelli, E., & Dragone, . (1994). Ureteral jet during medical treatment of benign prostatic hypertrophy. Arch Ital Urol Androl., 66, 45-8.

[68] Sperandeo, M., Sperandeo, G., Carella, M., Bianco, G., Cera, A., & Scarale, M. G. (1996). Ureteral jet in patients with benign prostatic hypertrophy: prognostic evaluation during single and combined therapy. Arch Ital Urol Androl., 68, 175-8.

[69] Stephens, F. D., & Lenaghan, D. (1962). The anatomical basis and dynamics of vesicoureteral reflux. J Urol., 87, 669-80.

[70] Stewart, J. C. (1937). On the mechanism of the uretero-vesical sphincter. Quart J Exp Physiol., 27, 193-204.

[71] Summers, R. M., Adler, R. S., Fowlkes, J. B., & Rubin, J. M. (1992). Laminar Submerged Jets by Color Doppler Ultrasound. A Model of the Ureteral Jet Phenomenon. Invest Radiol., 27, 1044-51.

[72] Sweet, C. S., Silbergleit, R., & Sanders, W. P. (1995). MRI demonstration of ureteral jet effect in a patient with a spinal ganglioneuroma. Pediatr Radiol., 25, 574-5.

[73] Tal, Z., Jaffe, H., Rosenak, D., Nadjari, M., & Hornstein, E. (1994). Ureteric jet examination by color Doppler ultrasound versus IVP for the assessment of ureteric patency following pelvic surgery-a pilot study. Eur J Obstet Gynecol Reprod Biol., 54, 119-22.

[74] Tanagho, E. A. (2000). Ch 1 Anatomy of the Genitourinary Tract In Tanagho EA et al ed Smith's General Urology. Lange Medical Books/McGraw Hill.

[75] Tanagho, E. A., Meyers, F. H., & Smith, D. R. (1968). The trigone: anatomical and physiological considerations. 1 In relation to the ureterovesical junction. J Urol. , 100, 623-32.

[76] Tanagho, E. A., & Pugh, R. C. B. (1963). The anatomy and function of the ureterovesical junction. Br J Urol., 35, 151-65.

[77] Timor-Tritsch, I. E., Haratz-Rubinstein, N., Monteagudo, A., Lerner, J. P., & Murphy, K. E. (1997). Transvaginal Color Doppler Sonography of the Ureteral Jets: A Method to Detect Ureteral Patency. Obstet Gynecol., 89, 113-7.

[78] Versari, R. (1908). Sur le developpement de la tunique musculaire de la vessie et particulierement sur le developement de la musculature du trigone et du sphincter a fibres lisses. Ann des Mal des Org Genito-Urin.26:561.

[79] Wachsberg, R. H. (1998). Unilateral Absence of Ureteral Jets in the Third Trimester of Pregnancy: Pitfall in Color Doppler US Diagnosis of Urinary Obstruction. Radiology., 209, 279-81.

[80] Waldeyer, W. (1892). Ureterscheide, Verhandl. Anat Gesellsch., 6, 259-61.

[81] Wu, C. C., Yao, W. J., Lin Jr, F., Hsieh, H. L., & Hwang, M. H. (1995). Spectral Analysis of Ureteral Jets by Color Doppler Ultrasonography: A Preliminary Uretero- Dynamic Study. J Med Ultrasound., 3, 64-9.

[82] Yoon, D. Y., Bae, S. H., & Choi, C. S. (2000). Transrectal Ultrasonography of Distal Ureteral Calculi: Comparison with Intravenous Urography. J Ultrasound Med. , 19, 271-5.

[83] Zaffagnini, B., & Mangiaracina, A. (1955). Premesse morfologiche alla dinamica della porzione terminale dell'uretere. Chir e patol sper.3:211.

Section 3

Genetical and Immunological Implications for Urinary Tract Infections

Chapter 7

Genetic Factors Underlying Susceptibility to Acute Pyelonephritis and Post-infectious Renal Damage

Maja Zivkovic, Ljiljana Stojkovic,
Brankica Spasojevic-Dimitrijeva, Mirjana Kostic and
Aleksandra Stankovic

Additional information is available at the end of the chapter

http://dx.doi.org/10.5772/52852

1. Introduction

Urinary tract infections (UTIs) are significant problem in infants and children and may be associated with renal scarring, which can cause serious long-term complications particularly hypertension and renal failure. The common characteristic of all UTIs is a significant growth of bacteria in the urinary tract. Uropathogenic Escherichia coli (*E. coli*) is the primary causative agent of UTIs.

Symptomatic UTIs can be classified into infections limited to the lower urinary tract and infections of the upper urinary tract. Marked individual differences in susceptibility to UTIs have been known for decades. Through different molecular interactions bacteria may trigger epithelial cell responses, cause cell detachment and invade or kill cells by apoptosis. The individual inflammatory response determines severity of acute pyelonephritis (APN) as well as differences in response to UTI among individuals. It is suggested that APN occurs more readily in high responders. Level of individual inflammatory response could be a key of enigma why some patients with APN develop renal scarring and progressive kidney damage whereas others do not.

Identification of new markers underlying APN and affecting its treatment is essential for designing interventions that would minimize tissue damage. Research of individual genetic background of inflammatory response suggests the significance of proinflammatory cytokine genes and polymorphisms of these genes. Such polymorphisms can occur either in regulatory or in coding regions of genes. They may affect the level of inflammation by enhancing transcription of certain cytokines' genes and thus increasing production of these cytokines. Changes in genes' expression as well as presence of certain alleles associated with disease phenotype support the hypothesis that genetic factors could modify susceptibility to acute pyelonephritis and post-infectious renal damage.

Several mechanical forces including urine flow and voiding, mucus shedding, and epithelial cell sloughing are important in minimizing UTI incidence. Bacterial adherence to the epithelium triggers defense responses. One of these is innate immunity response, which is important for uropathogenic *E. coli* recognition and immunomobilization. The innate immunity response is mediated by toll-like receptors (TLR4, TLR5, TLR11), adhesion molecules (E-selectin, ICAM-1, PECAM-1) and secreted factors such as cytokines (TNF-alpha, IL-1beta, IL-6, G-CSF, IL-17) and chemokines (CXCL1, CXCL2, CXCL3, CXCL8, CCL4). These molecules have been detected in mammalian bladder upon infection. Therefore, polymorphisms in genes coding for these molecules have been recognized as genetic susceptibility factors for UTIs. Neutrophils are the most abundant early responders to infection, while the antigen(Ag)-presenting macrophages, dendritic cells and innate-like lymphocytes (such as gamma delta T cells) have been implicated in the UTI host defense.

The cytokine response is essential for antibacterial defense of the urinary tract. Interleukin-8 (IL-8) is a potent chemoattractant responsible for neutrophil infiltration into the urinary tract. It was reported that neutrophils of children with recurrent pyelonephritis had lower expression of IL-8 receptor (CXCR1) than neutrophils of healthy controls. Interleukin-6 (IL-6) is one of the pro-inflammatory cytokines, which stimulates production of all acute-phase proteins thus contributing to acute-phase response and systemic inflammation. High serum or urine levels of IL-6 have been found in children with UTIs, particularly in children with APN compared to those with lower UTI. It was also indicated that urine and serum levels of cytokines could be observed as markers of renal damage as well as tools for monitoring the development and outcome of APN. Urine analysis has been extensively used by clinicians to diagnose various renal diseases. Advances in technology of molecular biology enable analyses of genes' expression levels in urine sediment. These expression studies have a potential to improve the diagnosis of APN by detecting urinary gene expression profiles, which are specific for patients with APN.

Besides susceptibility to UTIs, of great therapeutic importance is susceptibility to post-infectious renal damage in APN patients. This kidney damage susceptibility has the genetic component. Among the candidate genes are those coding for molecules like growth factors (TGF-β1, VEGF), which play important roles in processes characteristic for the tissue damage and scarring such as cell proliferation and accumulation of extracellular matrix. Angiotensin II, main effector of the renin-angiotensin system, is also considered a growth factor involved in all phenomena of renal tissue damaging and scar formation.

Here we will review the roles of candidate genes' polymorphisms and expression in susceptibility to APN and post-infectious renal scarring, in order to summarize the existing results and point out to further possible directions for research in this field.

2. Acute Pyelonephritis (APN) in children and genetic susceptibility to APN

Urinary tract infections (UTIs) are common among children of all ages including infants. UTI is defined as a penetration of microorganisms, mainly *E. coli*, into the tissue of urinary tract, which is marked by significant bacteriuria (>10^5 bacteria per 1ml of urine) [1]. UTIs are classified into three categories: upper UTI- acute pyelonephritis, lower UTI-acute cystitis and asymptomatic bacteriuria (ABU). The upper UTI, or acute pyelonephritis (APN), represents bacterial infection of renal parenchyma, which may cause various inflammatory lesions. Post-infectious renal scarring is the most serious complication following APN in children, with an estimated incidence of 10-65% [1-2]. Vesico-ureteral reflux (VUR) may also play an important role in renal damage [3]. VUR is suggested to be a weak predictor of permanent renal damage in children hospitalized with UTI [4] but it is also known that the grade of VUR positively correlates with likelihood of renal scarring [5]. Extensive renal scarring leads to renal insufficiency and hypertension [6-7]. Early diagnosis of APN and follow up to identify renal scarring after the first APN are thus very important. The primary distinction of APN is based on clinical manifestations and indirect laboratory testing of inflammatory markers such as C-reactive protein (CRP) serum levels, peripheral white blood cells' (WBC) count etc. However, these tests are unreliable in acute phase of pyelonephritis. The ^{99m}Tc-dimercaptosuccinic acid (DMSA) scintigraphy is a golden standard method for detection of acute renal inflammatory lesions specific for diagnosis of APN as well as for the follow-up detection of renal cortical scars [8-9]. Detection of permanent renal parenchymal defects following APN is ultimate for long-term prognosis of kidney function. The incidence of renal defects correlates inversely with the time interval between pyelonephritis and the scintigraphic study and stabilizes 4-6 months following acute disease. DMSA scintigraphy is based on binding of 99mTc-DMSA to renal parenchyma cells and therefore provides means of distinguishing APN from lower UTI and evaluating persistent DMSA uptake defects after the initial infection in children [8-10]. Given that DMSA exposes the patients to radiation, this procedure is not regularly used to diagnose APN.

2.1. Bacterial virulence and uroepithelial contact

Uropathogenic *Escherichia coli* is the most common causative agent (80%) of uncomplicated UTIs although other enteric organisms have been identified as well [11]. After colonization of the urethra and ascent to the bladder, bacteria bind to glycosphingolipid and glycoprotein receptors on the urinary tract epithelium and penetrate into tissue of urinary tract [12]. They express a number of virulence determinants that contribute to successful colonization of the urinary tract [13]. Many pathogenic microorganisms use host cell surface oligosaccharides including glycosphingolipids (GSLs) as receptors to attach to uroepithelial cells. The attachment of *E. coli* is mediated trough expression of flagellin and ascending of *E. coli* to the upper urinary tract and dissemination of bacteria within the host are enabled through a flagellum-mediated motility [14-16]. These actions, along with the lipid A moiety of lipopolysaccharide (endotoxin), have been shown to enhance activation of the host inflammatory response. Cytokines mediate this response [7,17-19]. Neutrophils are the first cells that migrate to the uroepithelium in the event of UTI and they are crucial in control of infection at early time points [20].

2.2. Renal scarring following APN

Bacterial infection of renal parenchyma during APN represents the major cause of acquired renal damage in children. The inflammatory changes associated with acute pyelonephritis are reversible but in some cases they result in renal defects. The percentage of children with renal scarring detected six months after the first APN is similar in the recent studies [21-23] and is in agreement with the results of European meta-analysis study of post-pyelonephritic renal scarring incidence [24]. Post-infectious renal scarring, as the most serious complication following APN, appears in 10-65% of children [8,25]. This renal damage can lead to hypertension and chronic renal failure [26-28].

The actual etiology of renal scarring remains controversial. The risk factors supposed to be associated with renal scars are: presence of vesico-ureteral reflux (VUR), delay in adequate antibiotic treatment, presence of recurrent UTI, bacterial virulence, host defense factors, host inflammatory and immunologic reactions and genetic susceptibility.

2.3. Vesico-Ureteral Reflux (VUR) as a risk factor for renal scarring

VUR is classically considered a risk factor for development of renal scars. The theory that reflux might play an important role in renal damage was proposed by Hodson and Edvards in 1960 [29]. Ransley and Risdon showed that scarring occurred only when urinary infection was present in association with VUR and intrarenal reflux [30]. Later it was suggested that VUR was a weak predictor of permanent renal damage in children hospitalized with UTI [31]. However, development of scars occurred even in absence of VUR, so there has been a debate for many years over the role of VUR in children who developed renal scars following UTI [31-35]. There is also a debate whether the grade of VUR positively correlates with likelihood of renal scarring or not [36] and whether the age represents a risk factor for scars' formation [37]. Gleeson and Gordon reported that there was a significant correlation between detection of a scarred kidney on DMSA scan and presence of VUR in children who were less than one year old [37]. In children aged over one year there was a poor correlation with renal scarring, so they suggested that the young growing kidney might be more vulnerable to insults. However, others [25,38-39] did not confirm that younger children were at greater risk for development of renal sequelae following pyelonephritis. Moreover, in some studies [40] children aged over one year had a higher frequency of renal scarring in comparison to infants.

2.4. Host inflammatory response and kidney damage following APN

Roberts et al. have suggested that the acute inflammatory response causing the eradication of bacteria could be responsible for the early pyelonephritic damage of renal tissue and subsequent renal scarring [41]. Neutrophils migrate between tissue compartments and exert their effector functions at different sites. They circulate in blood and interact with the endothelial lining that they cross to reach peripheral tissues. There is increasing evidence that the fate of neutrophils outside the vascular system is governed by specialized molecular interactions distinct from those in blood vessels [3] but these aspects have received less attention and are not well understood. Mucosal pathogens trigger a rapid neutrophil response [4-5], given that neutrophils are crucial effectors of the host defense [6-7]. The mucosal neutrophil response initiates when bacteria stimulate the epithelial cells to secrete chemokines [5,42] and to increase their chemokine receptors' expression. Neutrophils respond to so-formed chemotactic gradient, leave the bloodstream, travel through the submucosa and reach the basal side of the epithelial barrier, which they cross into the lumen [3,42]. Attention has been focused on molecular interactions of neutrophils with endothelial cells during the extravasation process [1-2], because this is the key to subsequent pathology and tissue destruction.

2.5. Genetic susceptibility to APN and renal scarring following APN

The interindividual differences in frequency and severity of UTIs exist and they are consistent with a genetic predisposition among disease-prone individuals. Structural defects such as congenital anomalies of kidney and urinary tract as well as social and environmental factors influence disease susceptibility [1-2]. There have been many attempts to identify the host factors that predispose to UTIs, especially to acute pyelonephritis (APN). Recurrent APN occurs within a small group of highly susceptible individuals, some of whom develop progressive renal scarring and therefore may need dialysis or kidney transplantation [2-4].

In an attempt to characterize the critical mechanisms and candidate genes for APN susceptibility, the "knockout" mice were investigated. It has been shown that the innate immunity response genes strongly influence susceptibility to UTIs, particularly APN [5-7].

Large interindividual differences both in frequency and severity of UTIs are consistent with genetic predisposition among disease-prone individuals although inherited defects in mechanisms of defense against UTIs have not been identified. Since the experimental studies suggested that susceptibility to clinical APN was genetically controlled and that the disease severity might vary with the expression levels of specific host response molecules, the next step was to investigate the susceptibility candidate genes in human population.

2.5.1. Cytokines

Phagocytosis of microorganisms and their intracellular degradation by the tissue macrophages represent stimuli for synthesis of proinflammatory cytokines, interleukin-1 (IL-1) and tumor necrosis factor-alpha (TNF-α) [43]. IL-1 and TNF-α induce expression of the adhesion molecules on the surface of endothelial cells, which bind the circulating leukocytes and allow their recruitment into the tissue. IL-1 and TNF-α also stimulate cells of the infected tissue to produce other mediators of inflammation such as cytokine interleukin-6 (IL-6) and chemokines, which regulate leukocytes' functions as well as their transendothelial migration into the inflammatory tissue [43]. Chemokines, particularly interleukin-8 (IL-8), are released from stimulated endothelial cells and macrophages. They act as chemoattractants stimulating the chemotaxis of neutrophils and neutrophil adhesion to stimulated endothelium [43,44].

Elevated serum levels of the proinflammatory cytokines- TNF-α, IL-1 and IL-6, have been measured in children with UTIs, with a significantly greater increase in children with APN than in those with lower UTI [10].

2.5.1.1. *TNF-α*

A single nucleotide polymorphism (SNP) -308 A/G in the promoter sequence of TNF-α gene is located at the binding site of the transcription factor activating protein-2 [45]. It has been suggested that TNF -308 A allele is related to a higher production of TNF-α [46]. No differences have been demonstrated in TNF-α -308 A/G genotype frequencies between infants with UTI (with and without renal scarring) and controls [47].

2.5.1.2. *IL-6*

Interleukin-6 (IL-6) is one of the pro-inflammatory cytokines, which stimulates production of all acute-phase proteins thus contributing to acute-phase response and systemic inflammation [10]. IL-6 is synthesized by several types of cells, in response to various antigens such as bacterial pathogens [48-49]. There are studies suggesting that IL-6 could be synthesized by uroepithelial or renal tubular cells [49-50]. High serum or urine levels of IL-6 have been detected in children with UTIs, particularly in those with APN in comparison to those with lower UTI [51-52]. It was indicated that urine and serum levels of this cytokine could be observed as markers of renal damage as well as tools for monitoring the development and outcome of APN [22,51-52].

Regulation of IL-6 expression is mainly accomplished at transcription level. A SNP -174 G/C, in the promoter region of IL-6 gene, is located 11 bp upstream from cis-regulatory element (CRE) and reported to influence the level of IL-6 expression in healthy individuals [53]. Moreover, -174 G/C polymorphism was found to be associated with circulating IL-6 levels and course of certain inflammatory diseases [54-55]. This polymorphism was investigated in association with APN and renal scarring in our study [21]. The genotype distributions and allele frequencies were not significantly different between the two investigated patients' groups, with APN and lower UTI. We concluded that IL-6 -174 G/C polymorphism was not a susceptibility factor for APN. This polymorphism was neither recognized as a risk factor for renal scarring in patients with the first APN [21]. Still, we detected a significant increase in white blood cells' count in APN children with CC genotype compared to those with wild type, GG, genotype.

2.5.1.3. *IL-8 and CXCR1*

The IL-8 receptor, CXCR1, was identified a candidate gene for acute pyelonephritis when mIL-8Rh mutant mice developed APN with severe tissue damage [6-7]. After sequencing that covered the entire CXCR1 gene two genetic variants, +217 C/G and +2608 G/C, were found to be susceptibility factors for APN in both children and adults [56]. Infants and children included in this study have been followed from their first episode of APN and adults had a history of APN in childhood. Kidney status was defined by DMSA scan. The UTI-associated CXCR1 variant, +217 C/G, has been shown to reduce RUNX1 binding to the putative intronic binding site. Furthermore, transfection experiments showed that transcription level of the mutant allele was lower, suggesting that +217 C/G polymorphism could reduce CXCR1 transcription [56].

The other study investigated polymorphisms of IL-8 gene, -251 A/T and +2767 A/G, and a polymorphism +2608 G/C of IL-8 receptor gene (CXCR1) in children with the first episode of upper UTI and APN documented by DMSA [18]. There were no statistically significant differences in genotype and allele frequencies of the IL-8 and CXCR1 polymorphisms between the UTI population and controls [18]. After comparison of genotype frequencies between DMSA positive children (with definite APN) and DMSA negative children, there were no significant differences between these two groups. Still, IL-8 -251 TT genotype was significantly more frequent in DMSA negative children suggesting that a carriage of A allele represents susceptibility factor for APN. By exclusion of patients with VUR, the genotype frequencies between DMSA positive and DMSA negative children were significantly different for IL-8 gene polymorphisms, -251 A/T and +2767 A/G. Again, -251 TT homozygotes were more frequent in DMSA negative children. These results, overall, suggest that IL-8 -251 A allele is significantly associated with presence of DMSA documented pyelonephritis [18]. Experimental data also showed that -251 A allele was associated with increase in IL-8 production in lipopolysaccharide stimulated whole blood [42]. The CXCR1 gene polymorphism +2608 G/C was not associated with APN [18].

2.5.1.4. MCP-1/CCL2 and RANTES/CCL5

Polymorphisms of genes coding for MCP-1 (monocyte chemotactic protein-1)/CCL2 and RANTES (Regulated upon Activation, Normal T-cell Expressed, and Secreted)/CCL5 and their receptors, CCR2 and CCR5 respectively, have been associated with the upper UTI. Only RANTES -403 G allele was significantly associated with risk for UTI, irrespectively of VUR [57].

2.5.2. Adhesion molecules

Initial steps of the inflammatory response are mediated by adhesion of inflammatory cells (leukocytes) to vascular endothelial cells [58-59]. Inflammatory cells then exit the circulation and infiltrate the surrounding tissue. This process is mediated by E-selectin, intercellular adhesion molecule-1 (ICAM-1) and platelet endothelial cell adhesion molecule-1 (PECAM-1) through the sequential steps of rolling, strong adhesion and diapedesis, respectively [59-60]. Data from ICAM-1 knockout animals showed that these animals had elevated neutrophil and lymphocyte counts and decreased neutrophil influx to the site of infection [61].

In the group of children with a proven history of UTI, E-selectin, ICAM-1, PECAM-1 and CD11b gene polymorphisms were investigated. There were no significant differences in allele frequencies between patients and controls for any of the investigated polymorphisms

[62]. Still, A allele of ICAM-1 exon 4 (G/A) polymorphism had significantly lower frequency in patients who developed renal scars following UTI compared with the patients without scars. This suggested that the A allele might be a protective factor for renal scarring following UTI. It is possible that protective effect of the A allele on development of renal scars following UTI may be a result of decreased binding of neutrophils and other inflammatory cells to ICAM-1, resulting in reduced leukocyte infiltration and reduced tissue damage [62].

2.5.3. Toll-Like Receptors (TLRs)

Toll-like receptors' (TLRs) genes are among the most commonly studied in association with UTIs. Toll-like receptors are critical sensors of microbial attack and effectors of the TLR-dependent innate defense, which enables host to eliminate pathogens [63-65]. TLRs are located on the cell surface or within organelles, like phagosomes, and are involved in detection of microbial ligands such as flagellin (TLR5), lipopolysaccharide (TLR4) and bacterial lipopeptides (TLR1/2/6) [66].

Given that TLRs play a crucial role in the innate immune defense, their structures and functions are tightly regulated [67]. Numerous attempts have been made to identify TLRs structural genes' variations, which might be related to diseases. Structural gene polymorphisms are relatively rare [68] and their contributions to human diseases still remain unclear.

Recently, TLR4 gene promoter region has been shown considerably more variable than previously known [69]. It's been suggested that few genotype patterns might reflect selection for low-responder variants in the primary asymptomatic bacteriuria group, which might protect against severe UTI [69]. Previously, low TLR4 expression had mostly been attributed to tolerance and not to genetic variation affecting TLR4 expression. Recently, the first study proposing impact of TLR4 promoter genetic variants on TLR4 expression has been published [69]. The authors have shown that single and multiple SNPs mostly suppressed TLR4 promoter activity *in vitro*, especially in response to *E. coli* infection. They have also observed that TLR4 promoter sequence variations could influence clinical presentation of UTI.

Hawn et al. [70] suggested that TLR4 Asp299Gly polymorphism was associated with protection from recurrent UTI, but not pyelonephritis. Furthermore, they showed that TLR5 +1174 C/T polymorphism was associated with an increased risk of recurrent UTI but not pyelonephritis, while a polymorphism in TLR1, +1805 G/T, was associated with protection from pyelonephritis in women [70]. The study that included children with recurrent UTI did not reveal a significant difference in Asp299Gly genotypes of TLR4 between children with UTI and control group [71].

Another study showed a relationship between the carrier status of HSPA1B (heat shock 70 kDa protein 1B) +1267 G and TLR4 +896 G alleles and development of recurrent UTI in childhood, independently on other urinary tract abnormalities [72]. Study in adults revealed that TLR4 +896 G allele had higher prevalence in UTI patients than in controls, and that TLR4 expression in monocytes was significantly lower in chronic UTI patients than in APN patients or healthy controls [73].

2.5.4. Vascular Endothelial Growth Factor (VEGF) and Transforming Growth Factor-beta1 (TGF-β1)

Vascular endothelial growth factor (VEGF) is a potent mitogen that enhances angiogenesis, microvascular permeability and proliferation of vascular endothelial cells [74]. Expression of VEGF has been detected in glomerular podocytes, epithelial cells of distal tubules and collecting ducts of kidney. Neovascularization in scarred kidney tissue and significant increase of urine VEGF levels associated with increased severity of renal scarring have been reported [75-76]. Transforming growth factor-beta1 (TGF-β1) appears to be one of the key factors in process of tissue repair. It is involved in regulation of cell proliferation, differentiation, extracellular matrix production and immune response [77]. Studies suggested that TGF-β1 could be involved in pathogenesis of congenital obstructive uropathies and renal scarring [78].

Several polymorphisms in VEGF and TGF-β1 genes have been linked to overproduction of these proteins as well as predisposition to progressive renal disease [79-81]. The VEGF -460 T/C polymorphism and TGF-β1 polymorphisms, -800 G/A and -509 C/T, have been associated with UTI and VUR in children [82]. VEGF -460 CC genotype was significantly more frequent in children with UTI and VUR than in controls [82]. Presence of VEGF -460 C allele increased basal VEGF promoter activity by 71% compared to the wild-type sequence [83]. Both UTI and VUR groups showed a significant increase in frequencies of TGF-β1 -800 GG and -509 CC genotypes in comparison to controls [82]. Cotton et al. [81] observed a correlation between -800 GA genotype and low TGF-β1 production *in vitro* suggesting a protective role against renal scarring. However, there was no correlation between TGF-β1 -509 genotypes and protein production [81].

In the study of Yim et al. [82], the UTI group was subdivided into two subgroups according to presence of renal scars. Significantly increased frequency of TGF-β1 +869 CC genotype was found in the subgroup of patients positive for renal scarring [82]. A study of nephropathy resulted in an association of the +869 CC genotype with heavy proteinuria and a higher score of mesangial cell proliferation [84].

2.5.5. Angiotensin I-Converting Enzyme (ACE)

Angiotensin II (Ang II), a powerful effector peptide of the renin-angiotensin system (RAS), is now considered a growth factor that plays active roles in all phenomena characteristic for renal tissue damage such as: proliferation of cells, accumulation of extracellular matrix and mononuclear cells' recruitment [19,85-87]. Since local kidney and interstitial fluid levels of Ang II are higher than the circulating [87], a blockade of Ang II actions may provide protection against functional and structural kidney deterioration.

Angiotensin I-converting enzyme (ACE), representing a target for ACE inhibitors (ACEI), is the key enzyme of RAS system. An insertion/deletion (I/D) polymorphism resulting from the presence/absence of a 287 bp *Alu* sequence has been identified in intron 16 of ACE gene [88-89]. This polymorphic variation in ACE gene correlates with levels of both circulating

[88] and tissue-localized ACE [90] and DD genotype is found to be associated with the highest ACE levels.

Gene polymorphisms of the RAS, especially I/D polymorphism of ACE gene, were associated with development of renal scarring in patients with congenital urological abnormalities [91-95]. It was concluded that the DD genotype could be a genetic susceptibility factor contributing to renal parenchymal damage. In our previous study [96], we found a difference in ACE I/D genotypes' distribution in patients with bladder dysfunction according to presence/absence of renal scarring. Although the two groups of patients (with and without scarring) did not differ by conventional risk factors, significant increase of D allele frequency was present in patients with renal scarring [96]. Only few studies investigated effect of ACE I/D polymorphism on renal scarring following APN. In Korean children frequencies of ACE I/D genotypes and alleles were not different between renal scar-positive and scar-negative groups, irrespectively of VUR [97]. Another study in Greek population did not confirm a correlation between ACE DD genotype and renal scar formation in children with UTIs [98].

2.5.6. Meta-analysis of genetic susceptibility factors for renal scar formation following UTI

Recently, meta-analysis of candidate gene polymorphisms as genetic susceptibility factors for renal scars' formation following UTI has been performed [99]. After systematic analysis of previously published data, the authors made strict inclusion criteria for this meta-analysis. From 523 original citations they identified only 18 articles that met the inclusion criteria. The results of meta-analysis showed that, according to recessive model of inheritance, ACE I/D polymorphism was a significant risk factor for renal scarring although with a high degree of between-study variability. According to dominant model, the T allele of TGF-β1 -509 C/T polymorphism was related to increased susceptibility for renal scarring, again with a high degree of between-study variability [99].

The risk for renal scarring occurred in ACE DD genotype carriers [99]. This genotype was correlated with increased expression of renal ACE [100] and thus with increased production of Ang II. Ang II is a mediator of progressive renal failure [101] and it may induce expression of TGF-β1, which is involved in pathogenesis of renal scarring [78,102]. There was no correlation found between TGF-β1 -509 genotypes and TGF-β1 protein production [81]. Considering the results of current meta-analysis [99] and known effects of ACE I/D polymorphism [100], it is of interest to study the effects of TGF-β1 -509 C/T gene polymorphism on gene expression and TGF-β1 levels in renal tissue of UTI (APN) patients having renal scars.

3. Conclusions

The symptoms of urinary tract infections (UTIs) depend on localization of infection and magnitude of the host response to bacteria. There are many risk factors for UTIs such as gender, VUR, environmental and socio-economical factors and, as it is proposed and reviewed here, genetic risk factors. Hence, UTIs represent a classical example of multifactorial disease

http://dx.doi.org/10.5772/52852

combining gene-environment and probably gene-gene interactions. To date, association with UTIs has been studied through a candidate gene approach. Among the candidate genes are those that code for soluble mediators, receptors and adhesion molecules included in regulation of the host response upon UTI. There are two basic approaches in these genetic studies. The first approach, which is less common, involves investigation of the candidate genes' effects on UTI susceptibility only (case-control study design). The second, more common approach, is based on investigation of susceptibility to renal scarring as the most serious complication of UTI (case study design). The second approach has a greater clinical potential since the primary aim of such research is to identify the patients susceptible to progressive kidney damage, which often results in end-stage renal disease.

The field investigating genetic susceptibility to UTIs in humans started only a decade ago as we can see from the reviewed articles. The first evidence that susceptibility to APN as well as asymptomatic bacteriuria (ABU) could be inherited came only a few years ago [69,103]. As a consequence, limited number of studies has been performed. Most of these studies included children only, some of the rest included both children and adults, while others included adults only. This review is focused on studies in children. Besides the number of studies, another limitation of research in this field is the number of participants included in these studies. The majority of studies reviewed here had about 100 patients, only few had up to 250. In further analysis of study design we must notice dividing of patients' group in subgroups- those with APN and those with lower UTI, and further dividing of the APN subgroup according to presence/absence of renal scarring. These limitations must be minimized in order to improve the statistical power of studies. Nevertheless, the results so far support the hypothesis of genetic impact on susceptibility to UTI/APN and give a good reason for further research.

Among genes mostly investigated in susceptibility to UTIs are the cytokine family genes. Results suggest that IL-8 -251 A allele represents a risk factor for APN, after exclusion of patients with VUR [18]. Single base changes in IL-8 receptor (CXCR1) gene, +217 C/G and +2608 G/C, are associated with a risk for APN in both children and adults [56]. RANTES/CCL5 -403 G allele is susceptibility factor for UTI, irrespectively of VUR [57].

The effects of TLRs genes' polymorphisms are hard to summarize due to a large number of genes and polymorphisms in this family and a small number of homogenous studies. It is proposed that genetic variants in TLR4 promoter influence TLR4 expression as well as clinical presentation of UTI [69]. Probably the most intereting, recent findings are the results of the group from Lundt University. Children with ABU express less TLR4 than APN prone children or controls but do not carry structural gene mutations explaining this phenotype. They recently defined the eight TLR4 promoter sequence variants, forming 19 haplotypes and 29 genotype patterns. The ABU-associated genotypes reduced TLR4 expression and the response to infection [56, 69]. Host susceptibility to common infections like UTI may thus be strongly influenced by single gene modifications affecting the innate immune response. For example, genetic alterations that reduce TLR4 function are associated with ABU, while polymorphisms reducing IRF3 or CXCR1 expression are associated with acute pyelonephritis and an increased risk for renal scarring [104]. The TLR1 +1805 G/T polymorphism is shown to protect against pyelonephritis in women [70]. It seems plausible to personalize the diagnosis and therapy of APN and ABU in the future, by combining information on bacterial virulence and the host response

To assess the genetic basis of renal scarring following UTI, many risk factors have to be analyzed. As we discussed, the heterogeneity between studies is large. Therefore, we may only point out to results of recent meta-analysis. The meta-analysis reveals that ACE I/D and TGF-β1 -509 C/T polymorphisms are risk factors for development of renal scars following UTI [99].

The most recent results strongly suggest the innate immunity as possible key factor for genetic susceptibility to APN and renal scarring after infection, although on murine models in which certan genes are functionaly similar to humans. It was shown that acute pyelonephritis and renal scarring are caused by dysfunctional innate immunity in mCxcr2 heterozygous mice [105].

Up to date no genome-wide association study has been done to use new approach for discovering novel genetic susceptibility factors for UTIs on a large number of individuals. New approaches to risk assasment and therapy shoud be encouraged and it is time for UTI to combine molecular medicine and social and behaviral factors. It is certain that some children are protected from APN and others prone to severe and recurent infections. Also, some of the gene polymorphisms are differentialy presented in those groups of children., The final aim is to identify the patients genetically susceptible to renal scarring and to discover and enable novel strategies in management of recurrent UTIs in order to prevent further renal damage especially in susceptible children. Until then, the prophylactic antibiotic treatment to prevent recurrent UTIs remains of limited usefulness [106].

Acknowledgement

This work is supported by Serbian Ministry of Education and Science Grant 175085.

Author details

Maja Zivkovic[1], Ljiljana Stojkovic[1], Brankica Spasojevic-Dimitrijeva[2], Mirjana Kostic[2] and Aleksandra Stankovic[1]

*Address all correspondence to: alexas@vinca.rs

1 Laboratory for Radiobiology and Molecular Genetics, "Vinca" Institute of Nuclear Sciences, University of Belgrade, Belgrade, Serbia

2 Nephrology Department, University Children's Hospital, School of Medicine, University of Belgrade, Belgrade, Serbia

References

[1] Kunin C. Urinary Tract Infections: Detection, Prevention and Management. Baltimore: Lippincott Williams & Wilkins; 1997.

[2] Stamm WE, McKevitt M, Roberts PL, White NJ. Natural history of recurrent urinary tract infections in women. Reviews of Infectious Diseases 1991;13: 77-84. http://www.jstor.org/stable/4455768

[3] Hodson CJ, Maling TM, McManamon PJ, Lewis MG. The Pathogenesis of Reflux Nephropathy (Chronic Atrophic Pyelonephritis). British Journal of Radiology Supplement 1975;13 1-26.

[4] Ransley PG, Risdon RA. Reflux and Renal Scarring. British Journal of Radiology Supplement 1978;14 1-38.

[5] Hagberg L, Briles DE, Eden CS. Evidence for separate genetic defects in C3H/HeJ and C3HeB/FeJ mice, that affect susceptibility to gram-negative infections. Journal of Immunology 1985;134(6): 4118-22. http://www.jimmunol.org/content/134/6/4118.long

[6] Hang L, Frendeus B, Godaly G, Svanborg C. Interleukin-8 receptor knockout mice have subepithelial neutrophil entrapment and renal scarring following acute pyelonephritis. Journal of Infectious Diseases 2000;182(6): 1738-48. http://jid.oxfordjournals.org/content/182/6/1738.long

[7] Frendeus B, Godaly G, Hang L, Karpman D, Lundstedt AC, Svanborg C. Interleukin 8 receptor deficiency confers susceptibility to acute experimental pyelonephritis and may have a human counterpart. Journal of Experimental Medicine 2000;192(6): 881-90. http://jem.rupress.org/content/192/6/881.long

[8] Rushton HG. The evaluation of acute pyelonephritis and renal scarring with technetium 99m-dimercaptosuccinic acid renal scintigraphy: evolving concepts and future directions. Pediatric Nephrology 1997;11(1): 108-20. http://www.springerlink.com/content/1t6wlqm1gkrxyny3/

[9] Biggi A, Dardanelli L, Pomero G, Cussino P, Noello C, Sernia O, Spada A. Camuzzini G. Acute renal cortical scintigraphy in children with a first urinary tract infection. Pediatric Nephrology 2001;16(9): 733-8. http://www.springerlink.com/content/2m7tq3525ltwb97d/

[10] Gürgöze MK, Akarsu S, Yilmaz E, Gödekmerdan A, Akça Z, Ciftçi I, Aygün AD. Proinflammatory cytokines and procalcitonin in children with acute pyelonephritis. Pediatric Nephrology 2005;20(10): 1445-8. http://www.springerlink.com/content/q32254407676682n/

[11] Foxman B, Barlow R, D'Arcy H, Gillespie B, Sobel JD. Urinary tract infection: self-reported incidence and associated costs. Annals of Epidemiology 2000;10(8): 509-15. http://www.annalsofepidemiology.org/article/S1047-2797(00)00072-7/fulltext

[12] Lambert H., Coulthard M. The Child with Urinary Tract Infection. In: Lambert H., Coulthard M. (3rd ed.) Clinical Paediatric Nephrology. Oxford: Oxford University Press; 2003. p197-225.

[13] Johnson JR. Virulence factors in Escherichia coli urinary tract infection. Clinical Microbiology Reviews 1991;4(1): 80-128. http://cmr.asm.org/content/4/1/80.long

[14] Lane MC, Alteri CJ, Smith SN, Mobley HL. Expression of flagella is coincident with uropathogenic Escherichia coli ascension to the upper urinary tract. Proceedings of the National Academy of Sciences of the United States of America 2007;104(42): 16669-74. http://www.pnas.org/content/104/42/16669.long

[15] Leffler H, Edén SC. Chemical identification of a glycosphingolipid receptor for Escherichia coli attaching to human urinary tract epithelial cells and agglutinating human erythrocytes. Federation of European Microbiological Societies Microbiology Letters 1980;8: 127-34. http://onlinelibrary.wiley.com/doi/10.1111/j.1574-6968.1980.tb05064.x/pdf

[16] Svensson M, Platt F, Frendeus B, Butters T, Dwek R, Svanborg C. Carbohydrate receptor depletion as an antimicrobial strategy for prevention of urinary tract infection. Journal of Infectious Diseases 2001;183(1): S70-3. http://jid.oxfordjournals.org/content/183/Supplement_1/S70.long

[17] Kassir K, Vargas-Shiraishi O, Zaldivar F, Berman M, Singh J, Arrieta A. Cytokine profiles of pediatric patients treated with antibiotics for pyelonephritis: potential therapeutic impact. Clinical and Vaccine Immunology 2001;8(6): 1060-3. http://cvi.asm.org/content/8/6/1060.long

[18] Artifoni L, Negrisolo S, Montini G, Zucchetta P, Molinari PP, Cassar W, Destro R, Anglani F, Rigamonti W, Zacchello G, Murer L. Interleukin-8 and CXCR1 receptor functional polymorphisms and susceptibility to acute pyelonephritis. Journal of Urology 2007;177(3): 1102-6. http://www.jurology.com/article/S0022-5347(06)02763-7/fulltext

[19] Klahr S, Schreiner G, Ichikawa I. The progression of renal disease. New England Journal of Medicine 1988;318(25): 1657-66. http://www.nejm.org/doi/full/10.1056/NEJM198806233182505

[20] Haraoka M, Hang L, Frendeus B, Godaly G, Burdick M, Strieter R, Svanborg C. Neutrophil recruitment and resistance to urinary tract infection. Journal of Infectious Diseases 1999;180(4): 1220-9. http://jid.oxfordjournals.org/content/180/4/1220.long

[21] Spasojević-Dimitrijeva B, Živković M, Stanković A, Stojković L, Kostić M. The IL-6 -174G/C polymorphism and renal scarring in children with first acute pyelonephritis. Pediatric Nephrology 2010;25(10): 2099-106. http://www.springerlink.com/content/fn0n1443032w4j14/

[22] Sheu JN, Chen MC, Chen SM, Chen SL, Chiou SY, Lue KH. Relationship between serum and urine interleukin-6 elevations and renal scarring in children with acute pye-

lonephritis. Scandinavian Journal of Urology and Nephrology 2009;43(2): 133-7. http://informahealthcare.com/doi/full/10.1080/00365590802478742

[23] Sheu JN, Chen MC, Cheng SL, Lee IC, Chen SM, Tsay GJ. Urine interleukin-1beta in children with acute pyelonephritis and renal scarring. Nephrology 2007;12(5): 487-93. http://onlinelibrary.wiley.com/doi/10.1111/j.1440-1797.2007.00819.x/full

[24] Faust WC, Diaz M, Pohl HG. Incidence of post-pyelonephritic renal scarring: a meta-analysis of the dimercapto-succinic acid literature. Journal of Urology 2009;181(1): 290-8. http://www.jurology.com/article/S0022-5347(08)02460-9/fulltext

[25] Stokland E, Hellstrom M, Jacobsson B, Jodal U, Sixt R. Renal damage one year after first urinary tract infection: role of dimercaptosuccinic acid scintigraphy. Journal of Pediatrics 1996;129(6): 815-20. http://www.jpeds.com/article/S0022-3476(96)70024-0/fulltext

[26] Lin DS, Huang SH, Lin CC, Tung YC, Huang TT, Chiu NC, Koa HA, Hung HY, Hsu CH, Hsieh WS, Yang DI, Huang FY. Urinary tract infection in febrile infants younger than eight weeks of Age. Pediatrics 2000;105(2): E20. http://pediatrics.aappublications.org/content/105/2/e20.long

[27] Jacobson SH, Hansson S, Jakobsson B. Vesico-ureteric reflux: occurrence and long-term risks. Acta Paediatrica Supplement 1999;88(431): 22-30. http://onlinelibrary.wiley.com/doi/10.1111/j.1651-2227.1999.tb01315.x/pdf

[28] Patzer L, Seeman T, Luck C, Wuhl E, Janda J, Misselwitz J. Day- and night-time blood pressure elevation in children with higher grades of renal scarring. Journal of Pediatrics 2003;142(2): 117-22. http://www.jpeds.com/article/S0022-3476(02)40215-6/fulltext

[29] Hodson CJ, Edwards D. Chronic pyelonephritis and vesico-ureteric reflex. Clinical Radiology 1960;11: 219-31. http://www.sciencedirect.com/science/article/pii/S0009926060800475

[30] Ransley PG, Risdon RA. Renal papillary morphology and intrarenal reflux in the young pig. Urological Research 1975;3(3): 105-9. https://springerlink3.metapress.com/content/76tx50l4104m205l/resource-secured/?target=fulltext.pdf&sid=2ufmjss-pu0cpf0s2zqqlkv3l&sh=www.springerlink.com

[31] Gordon I, Barkovics M, Pindoria S, Cole TJ, Woolf AS. Primary vesicoureteric reflux as a predictor of renal damage in children hospitalized with urinary tract infection: a systematic review and meta-analysis. Journal of the American Society of Nephrology 2003;14(3): 739-44. http://jasn.asnjournals.org/content/14/3/739.long

[32] Wheeler D, Vimalachandra D, Hodson EM, Roy LP, Smith G, Craig JC. Antibiotics and surgery for vesicoureteric reflux: a meta-analysis of randomised controlled trials. Archives of Disease in Childhood 2003;88(8): 688-94. http://adc.bmj.com/content/88/8/688.long

[33] Taskinen S, Ronnholm K. Post-pyelonephritic renal scars are not associated with vesicoureteral reflux in children. Journal of Urology 2005;173(4): 1345-8. http://www.jurology.com/article/S0022-5347(05)61098-1/fulltext

[34] Moorthy I, Easty M, McHugh K, Ridout D, Biassoni L, Gordon I. The presence of vesicoureteric reflux does not identify a population at risk for renal scarring following a first urinary tract infection. Archives of Disease in Childhood 2005;90(7): 733-6. http://adc.bmj.com/content/90/7/733.long

[35] Winberg J. Commentary: Progressive Renal Damage from Infection with or without Reflux. Journal of Urology 1992;148(5Pt2) 1733-1734.

[36] Preda I, Jodal U, Sixt R, Stokland E, Hansson S. Normal dimercaptosuccinic acid scintigraphy makes voiding cystourethrography unnecessary after urinary tract infection. Journal of Pediatrics 2007;151(6): 581-4. http://www.jpeds.com/article/S0022-3476(07)00457-X/fulltext

[37] Gleeson FV, Gordon I. Imaging in urinary tract infection. Archives of Disease in Childhood 1991;66(11): 1282-3. http://www.ncbi.nlm.nih.gov/pmc/articles/PMC1793291/pdf/archdisch00644-0022.pdf

[38] Rushton HG, Majd M, Jantausch B, Wiedermann BL, Belman AB. Renal Scarring Following Reflux and Nonreflux Pyelonephritis in Children: Evaluation with 99mTechnetium-Dimercaptosuccinic Acid Scintigraphy. Journal of Urology 1992;147(5) 1327-1332.

[39] Jakobsson B, Berg U, Svensson L. Renal scarring after acute pyelonephritis. Archives of Disease in Childhood 1994;70(2): 111-5. http://www.ncbi.nlm.nih.gov/pmc/articles/PMC1029711/

[40] Lee JH, Son CH, Lee MS, Park YS. Vesicoureteral reflux increases the risk of renal scars: a study of unilateral reflux. Pediatric nephrology 2006;21(9): 1281-4. https://springerlink3.metapress.com/content/k6670g573l638v10/resource-secured/?target=fulltext.html&sid=oqo3fxwy4viifcuku02qpzya&sh=www.springerlink.com

[41] Roberts JA, Domingue GJ, Martin LN, Kim JC. Immunology of pyelonephritis in the primate model: live versus heat-killed bacteria. Kidney International 1981;19(2): 297-305. http://www.nature.com/ki/journal/v19/n2/pdf/ki198120a.pdf

[42] Hull J, Ackerman H, Isles K, Usen S, Pinder M, Thomson A, Kwiatkowski D. Unusual haplotypic structure of IL8, a susceptibility locus for a common respiratory virus. American Journal of Human Genetics 2001;69(2): 413-9. http://www.sciencedirect.com/science/article/pii/S0002929707610866

[43] Abbas AK, Lichtman AH. Basic Immunology: Functions and Disorders of the Immune System. Philadelphia: WB Saunders; 2001.

[44] Glauser MP, Meylan P, Bille J. The inflammatory response and tissue damage. Pediatric Nephrology 1987;1(4): 615-22. https://springerlink3.metapress.com/content/

r160185l28762168/resource-secured/?target=fulltext.pdf&sid=oqo3fxwy4viifcu-ku02qpzya&sh=www.springerlink.com

[45] Brinkman BM, Giphart MJ, Verhoef A, Kaijzel EL, Naipal AM, Daha MR, Breedveld FC, Verweij CL. Tumor necrosis factor alpha-308 gene variants in relation to major histocompatibility complex alleles and Felty's syndrome. Hum Immunol. 1994;41(4): 259-66. http://www.sciencedirect.com/science/article/pii/0198885994900442

[46] Mayer FR, Messer G, Knabe W, Mempel W, Meurer M, Kolb HJ, Holler E. High Response of TNF Secretion in Vivo in Patients Undergoing BMT May be Associated with the 308 bp TNF-α Gene Enhancer Polymorphism. Bone Marrow Transplantation 1996;17 s101.

[47] Savvidou A, Bitsori M, Choumerianou DM, Karatzi M, Kalmanti M, Galanakis E. Polymorphisms of the TNF-alpha and ACE genes, and renal scarring in infants with urinary tract infection. Journal of Urology 2010;183(2): 684-7. http://www.jurology.com/article/S0022-5347(09)02666-4/fulltext

[48] Van-Snick J. Interleukin-6: an overview. Annual Review of Immunology 1990;8: 253-78. http://www.annualreviews.org/doi/pdf/10.1146/annurev.iy.08.040190.001345

[49] Curfs JH, Meis JF, Hoogkamp-Korstanje JA. A primer on cytokines: sources, receptors, effects, and inducers. Clinical Microbiology Reviews 1997;10(4): 742-80. http://cmr.asm.org/content/10/4/742.long

[50] Hedges S, Agace W, Svensson M, Sjogren AC, Ceska M, Svanborg C. Uroepithelial cells are part of a mucosal cytokine network. Infection and Immunity 1994;62(6): 2315-21. http://iai.asm.org/content/62/6/2315.long

[51] Roilides E, Papachristou F, Gioulekas E, Tsaparidou S, Karatzas N, Sotiriou J, Tsiouris J. Increased urine interleukin-6 concentrations correlate with pyelonephritic changes on 99mTc-dimercaptosuccinic acid scans in neonates with urinary tract infections. J Infect Dis. 1999;180(3): 904-7. http://jid.oxfordjournals.org/content/180/3/904.long

[52] Sheu JN, Chen MC, Lue KH, Cheng SL, Lee IC, Chen SM, Tsay GJ. Serum and urine levels of interleukin-6 and interleukin-8 in children with acute pyelonephritis. Cytokine 2006;36(5-6): 276-82. http://www.sciencedirect.com/science/article/pii/S1043466607000191

[53] Fishman D, Faulds G, Jeffery R, Mohamed-Ali V, Yudkin JS, Humphries S, Woo P. The effect of novel polymorphisms in the interleukin-6 (IL-6) gene on IL-6 transcription and plasma IL-6 levels, and an association with systemic-onset juvenile chronic arthritis. Journal of Clinical Investigation 1998;102(7): 1369-76. http://www.jci.org/articles/view/2629/pdf

[54] Bennet AM, Prince JA, Fei GZ, Lyrenas L, Huang Y, Wiman B, Frostegard J, Faire U. Interleukin-6 serum levels and genotypes influence the risk for myocardial infarc-

tion. Atherosclerosis 2003;171(2): 359-67. http://www.atherosclerosis-journal.com/article/S0021-9150(03)00392-7/fulltext

[55] Brull DJ, Montgomery HE, Sanders J, Dhamrait S, Luong L, Rumley A, Lowe GD, Humphries SE. Interleukin-6 gene -174g>c and -572g>c promoter polymorphisms are strong predictors of plasma interleukin-6 levels after coronary artery bypass surgery. Arteriosclerosis Thrombosis and Vascular Biology 2001;21(9): 1458-63. http://atvb.ahajournals.org/content/21/9/1458.long

[56] Lundstedt AC, McCarthy S, Gustafsson MC, Godaly G, Jodal U, Karpman D, Leijonhufvud I, Lindén C, Martinell J, Ragnarsdottir B, Samuelsson M, Truedsson L, Andersson B, Svanborg C. A genetic basis of susceptibility to acute pyelonephritis. Public Library of Science One 2007;2(9): e825. http://www.plosone.org/article/info%3Adoi%2F10.1371%2Fjournal.pone.0000825

[57] Centi S, Negrisolo S, Stefanic A, Benetti E, Cassar W, Da Dalt L, Rigamonti W, Zucchetta P, Montini G, Murer L, Artifoni L. Upper urinary tract infections are associated with RANTES promoter polymorphism. Journal of Pediatrics 2010;157(6): 1038-40. http://www.jpeds.com/article/S0022-3476(10)00674-8/fulltext

[58] Springer TA. Leucocyte adhesion to cells. Scandinavian Journal of Immunology 1990;32(3): 211-2. http://onlinelibrary.wiley.com/doi/10.1111/j.1365-3083.1990.tb02912.x/pdf

[59] Adams DH, Shaw S. Leucocyte-endothelial interactions and regulation of leucocyte migration. Lancet 1994;343(8901): 831-6. http://www.sciencedirect.com/science/article/pii/S014067369492029X

[60] Ross R. Atherosclerosis--an inflammatory disease. New England Journal of Medicine 1999;340(2): 115-26. http://www.nejm.org/doi/full/10.1056/NEJM199901143400207

[61] Xu H, Gonzalo JA, St Pierre Y, Williams IR, Kupper TS, Cotran RS, Springer TA, Gutierrez-Ramos JC. Leukocytosis and resistance to septic shock in intercellular adhesion molecule 1-deficient mice. Journal of Experimental Medicine 1994;180(1): 95-109. http://jem.rupress.org/content/180/1/95.long

[62] Gbadegesin RA, Cotton SA, Watson CJ, Brenchley PE, Webb NJ. Association between ICAM-1 Gly-Arg polymorphism and renal parenchymal scarring following childhood urinary tract infection. International Journal of Immunogenetics 2006;33(1): 49-53. http://onlinelibrary.wiley.com/doi/10.1111/j.1744-313X.2006.00565.x/full

[63] Poltorak A, He X, Smirnova I, Liu MY, Van Huffel C, Du X, Birdwell D, Alejos E, Silva M, Galanos C, Freudenberg M, Ricciardi-Castagnoli P, Layton B, Beutler B. Defective LPS signaling in C3H/HeJ and C57BL/10ScCr mice: mutations in Tlr4 gene. Science 1998;282(5396): 2085-8. http://www.sciencemag.org/content/282/5396/2085.full

[64] Iwasaki A, Medzhitov R. Toll-like receptor control of the adaptive immune responses. Nature Immunology 2004;5(10): 987-95. http://www.nature.com/ni/journal/v5/n10/full/ni1112.html

[65] Uematsu S, Akira S. Toll-like receptors and innate immunity. Journal of Molecular Medicine 2006;84(9): 712-25. https://springerlink3.metapress.com/content/l417556q5676u813/resource-secured/?target=fulltext.html&sid=jr1xcyn1vkolv5wazvustjnm&sh=www.springerlink.com

[66] Beutler B. Microbe sensing, positive feedback loops, and the pathogenesis of inflammatory diseases. Immunological Reviews 2009;227(1): 248-63. http://onlinelibrary.wiley.com/doi/10.1111/j.1600-065X.2008.00733.x/full

[67] Li X, Qin J. Modulation of Toll-interleukin 1 receptor mediated signaling. Journal of Molecular Medicine 2005;83(4): 258-66. https://springerlink3.metapress.com/content/eqb6dp9rcvqcfd62/resource-secured/?target=fulltext.html&sid=jr1xcyn1vkolv5wazvustjnm&sh=www.springerlink.com

[68] Smirnova I, Hamblin MT, McBride C, Beutler B, Di Rienzo A. Excess of rare amino acid polymorphisms in the Toll-like receptor 4 in humans. Genetics 2001;158(4): 1657-64. http://www.genetics.org/content/158/4/1657.long

[69] Ragnarsdottir B, Jonsson K, Urbano A, Gronberg-Hernandez J, Lutay N, Tammi M, Gustafsson M, Lundstedt AC, Leijonhufvud I, Karpman D, Wullt B, Truedsson L, Jodal U, Andersson B, Svanborg C. Toll-like receptor 4 promoter polymorphisms: common TLR4 variants may protect against severe urinary tract infection. Public Library of Science One. 2010;5(5): e10734. http://www.plosone.org/article/info%3Adoi%2F10.1371%2Fjournal.pone.0010734

[70] Hawn TR, Scholes D, Li SS, Wang H, Yang Y, Roberts PL, Stapleton AE, Janer M, Aderem A, Stamm WE, Zhao LP, Hooton TM. Toll-like receptor polymorphisms and susceptibility to urinary tract infections in adult women. Public Library of Science One 2009;4(6): e5990. http://www.plosone.org/article/info%3Adoi%2F10.1371%2Fjournal.pone.0005990

[71] Ertan P, Berdeli A, Yilmaz O, Gonulal DA, Yuksel H. LY96, UPKIB mutations and TLR4, CD14, MBL polymorphisms in children with urinary tract infection. Indian Journal of Pediatrics 2011;78(10): 1229-33. https://springerlink3.metapress.com/content/22300gq91150v807/resource-secured/?target=fulltext.html&sid=jr1xcyn1vkolv5wazvustjnm&sh=www.springerlink.com

[72] Karoly E, Fekete A, Banki NF, Szebeni B, Vannay A, Szabo AJ, Tulassay T, Reusz GS. Heat shock protein 72 (HSPA1B) gene polymorphism and Toll-like receptor (TLR) 4 mutation are associated with increased risk of urinary tract infection in children. Pediatric Research 2007;61(3): 371-4. http://www.nature.com/pr/journal/v61/n3/full/pr200773a.html

[73] Yin X, Hou T, Liu Y, Chen J, Yao Z, Ma C, Yang L, Wei L. Association of Toll-like receptor 4 gene polymorphism and expression with urinary tract infection types in

adults. Public Library of Science One 2010;5(12): e14223. http://www.plosone.org/article/info%3Adoi%2F10.1371%2Fjournal.pone.0014223

[74] Ferrara N, Chen H, Davis-Smyth T, Gerber HP, Nguyen TN, Peers D, Chisholm V, Hillan KJ, Schwall RH. Vascular endothelial growth factor is essential for corpus luteum angiogenesis. Nature Medicine 1998;4(3): 336-40. http://www.nature.com/nm/journal/v4/n3/pdf/nm0398-336.pdf

[75] Konda R, Sato H, Sakai K, Sato M, Orikasa S, Kimura N. Expression of platelet-derived endothelial cell growth factor and its potential role in up-regulation of angiogenesis in scarred kidneys secondary to urinary tract diseases. American Journal of Pathology 1999;155(5): 1587-97. http://linkinghub.elsevier.com/retrieve/pii/S0002-9440(10)65475-2

[76] Konda R, Sato H, Sakai K, Abe Y, Fujioka T. Urinary excretion of vascular endothelial growth factor is increased in children with reflux nephropathy. Nephron Clinical Practice 2004;98(3): c73-8. http://content.karger.com/ProdukteDB/produkte.asp?Aktion=ShowFulltext&ArtikelNr=000080676&Ausgabe=230425&ProduktNr=228539

[77] Border WA, Noble NA. Transforming growth factor beta in tissue fibrosis. New England Journal of Medicine 1994;331(19): 1286-92. http://www.nejm.org/doi/full/10.1056/NEJM199411103311907

[78] MacRae Dell K, Hoffman BB, Leonard MB, Ziyadeh FN, Schulman SL. Increased urinary transforming growth factor-beta(1) excretion in children with posterior urethral valves. Urology 2000;56(2): 311-4. http://www.goldjournal.net/article/S0090-4295(00)00591-4/fulltext

[79] Watson CJ, Webb NJ, Bottomley MJ, Brenchley PE. Identification of polymorphisms within the vascular endothelial growth factor (VEGF) gene: correlation with variation in VEGF protein production. Cytokine 2000;12(8): 1232-5. http://www.sciencedirect.com/science/article/pii/S1043466600906926

[80] Summers AM, Coupes BM, Brennan MF, Ralph SA, Short CD, Brenchley PE. VEGF -460 genotype plays an important role in progression to chronic kidney disease stage 5. Nephrology Dialysis Transplantation 2005;20(11): 2427-32. http://ndt.oxfordjournals.org/content/20/11/2427.long

[81] Cotton SA, Gbadegesin RA, Williams S, Brenchley PE, Webb NJ. Role of TGF-beta1 in renal parenchymal scarring following childhood urinary tract infection. Kidney International 2002;61(1): 61-7. http://www.nature.com/ki/journal/v61/n1/full/4492704a.html

[82] Yim HE, Bae IS, Yoo KH, Hong YS, Lee JW. Genetic control of VEGF and TGF-beta1 gene polymorphisms in childhood urinary tract infection and vesicoureteral reflux. Pediatric Research 2007;62(2): 183-7. http://www.nature.com/pr/journal/v62/n2/full/pr2007196a.html

[83] Stevens A, Soden J, Brenchley PE, Ralph S, Ray DW. Haplotype analysis of the polymorphic human vascular endothelial growth factor gene promoter. Cancer Research 2003;63(4): 812-6. http://cancerres.aacrjournals.org/content/63/4/812.long

[84] Sato F, Narita I, Goto S, Kondo D, Saito N, Ajiro J, Saga D, Ogawa A, Kadomura M, Akiyama F, Kaneko Y, Ueno M, Sakatsume M, Gejyo F. Transforming growth factor-beta1 gene polymorphism modifies the histological and clinical manifestations in Japanese patients with IgA nephropathy. Tissue Antigens 2004;64(1): 35-42. http://onlinelibrary.wiley.com/doi/10.1111/j.1399-0039.2004.00256.x/full

[85] Wolf G, Neilson EG. Angiotensin II as a renal growth factor. Journal of the American Society of Nephrology. 1993;3(9): 1531-40. http://jasn.asnjournals.org/content/3/9/1531.long

[86] Ruiz-Ortega M, Lorenzo O, Egido J. Angiotensin III up-regulates genes involved in kidney damage in mesangial cells and renal interstitial fibroblasts. Kidney International Supplement 1998;68: S41-5. http://www.nature.com/ki/journal/v54/n68s/full/4490546a.html

[87] Navar LG, Imig JD, Zou L, Wang CT. Intrarenal Production of Angiotensin II. Seminars in Nephrology 1997;17(5) 412-422.

[88] Rigat B, Hubert C, Alhenc-Gelas F, Cambien F, Corvol P, Soubrier F. An insertion/deletion polymorphism in the angiotensin I-converting enzyme gene accounting for half the variance of serum enzyme levels. Journal of Clinical Investigation 1990;86(4): 1343-6. http://www.jci.org/articles/view/114844

[89] Rigat B, Hubert C, Corvol P, Soubrier F. PCR detection of the insertion/deletion polymorphism of the human angiotensin converting enzyme gene (DCP1) (dipeptidyl carboxypeptidase 1). Nucleic Acids Research 1992;20(6): 1433. http://nar.oxfordjournals.org/content/20/6/1433.2.long

[90] Costerousse O, Allegrini J, Lopez M, Alhenc-Gelas F. Angiotensin I-converting enzyme in human circulating mononuclear cells: genetic polymorphism of expression in T-lymphocytes. Biochemical Journal 1993;290(1): 33-40. http://www.biochemj.org/bj/290/0033/2900033.pdf

[91] Hohenfellner K, Hunley TE, Brezinska R, Brodhag P, Shyr Y, Brenner W, Habermehl P, Kon V. ACE I/D gene polymorphism predicts renal damage in congenital uropathies. Pediatric Nephrology 1999;13(6): 514-8. https://springerlink3.metapress.com/content/jeqch0uu051pepu2/resource-secured/?target=fulltext.pdf&sid=hy1eoamsowpup4dwlzp21ept&sh=www.springerlink.com

[92] Al-Eisa A, Haider MZ, Srivastva BS. Angiotensin-converting enzyme gene insertion/deletion polymorphism and renal damage in childhood uropathies. Pediatrics International 2000;42(4): 348-53. http://onlinelibrary.wiley.com/doi/10.1046/j.1442-200x.2000.01242.x/full

[93] Haszon I, Friedman AL, Papp F, Bereczki C, Baji S, Bodrogi T, Karoly E, Endreffy E, Turi S. ACE gene polymorphism and renal scarring in primary vesicoureteric reflux. Pediatric Nephrology 2002;17(12): 1027-31. https://springerlink3.metapress.com/content/hf4xddgql6luh7yq/resource-secured/?target=fulltext.html&sid=hy1eoam-sowpup4dwlzp21ept&sh=www.springerlink.com

[94] Brock JW, 3rd, Adams M, Hunley T, Wada A, Trusler L, Kon V. Potential risk factors associated with progressive renal damage in childhood urological diseases: the role of angiotensin-converting enzyme gene polymorphism. Journal of Urology 1997;158(3 Pt 2): 1308-11. http://www.jurology.com/article/S0022-5347(01)64463-X/fulltext

[95] Ozen S, Alikasifoglu M, Saatci U, Bakkaloglu A, Besbas N, Kara N, Kocak H, Erbas B, Unsal I, Tuncbilek E. Implications of certain genetic polymorphisms in scarring in vesicoureteric reflux: importance of ACE polymorphism. American Journal of Kidney Diseases 1999;34(1): 140-5. http://www.sciencedirect.com/science/article/pii/S0272638699701204

[96] Kostić M, Stanković A, Živković M, Peco-Antić A, Jovanović O, Alavantić D, Kruscić D. ACE and AT1 receptor gene polymorphisms and renal scarring in urinary bladder dysfunction. Pediatric Nephrology 2004;19(8): 853-7. https://springerlink3.metapress.com/content/m0ln12arkyj52q0u/resource-secured/?target=fulltext.html&sid=5xlg00ojhmffszjl3yidz4up&sh=www.springerlink.com

[97] Cho SJ, Lee SJ. ACE gene polymorphism and renal scar in children with acute pyelonephritis. Pediatric Nephrology 2002;17(7): 491-5. https://springerlink3.metapress.com/content/wmr2ua8atbqqchg2/resource-secured/?target=fulltext.html&sid=5xlg00ojhmffszjl3yidz4up&sh=www.springerlink.com

[98] Sekerli E, Katsanidis D, Vavatsi N, Makedou A, Gatzola M. ACE gene insertion/deletion polymorphism and renal scarring in children with urinary tract infections. Pediatric Nephrology 2009;24(10): 1975-80. https://springerlink3.metapress.com/content/lw40768164675386/resource-secured/?target=fulltext.html&sid=5xlg00ojhmffszjl3yidz4up&sh=www.springerlink.com

[99] Zaffanello M, Tardivo S, Cataldi L, Fanos V, Biban P, Malerba G. Genetic susceptibility to renal scar formation after urinary tract infection: a systematic review and meta-analysis of candidate gene polymorphisms. Pediatric Nephrology 2011;26(7): 1017-29. https://springerlink3.metapress.com/content/2357371735545q41/resource-secured/?target=fulltext.html&sid=5xlg00ojhmffszjl3yidz4up&sh=www.springerlink.com

[100] Mizuiri S, Hemmi H, Kumanomidou H, Iwamoto M, Miyagi M, Sakai K, Aikawa A, Ohara T, Yamada K, Shimatake H, Hasegawa A. Angiotensin-converting enzyme (ACE) I/D genotype and renal ACE gene expression. Kidney International 2001;60(3): 1124-30. http://www.nature.com/ki/journal/v60/n3/full/4492521a.html

[101] Ishidoya S, Morrissey J, McCracken R, Reyes A, Klahr S. Angiotensin II receptor antagonist ameliorates renal tubulointerstitial fibrosis caused by unilateral ureteral ob-

struction. Kidney International 1995;47(5): 1285-94. http://www.nature.com/ki/journal/v47/n5/pdf/ki1995183a.pdf

[102] Pimentel JL, Sundell CL, Wang S, Kopp JB, Montero A, Martinez-Maldonado M. Role of angiotensin II in the expression and regulation of transforming growth factor-beta in obstructive nephropathy. Kidney International 1995;48(4): 1233-46. http://www.nature.com/ki/journal/v48/n4/pdf/ki1995407a.pdf

[103] Lundstedt AC, Leijonhufvud I, Ragnarsdottir B, Karpman D, Andersson B, Svanborg C. Inherited susceptibility to acute pyelonephritis: a family study of urinary tract infection. Journal of Infectious Diseases 2007;195(8): 1227-34. http://jid.oxfordjournals.org/content/195/8/1227.long

[104] Ragnarsdóttir B, Svanborg C. Susceptibility to acute pyelonephritis or asymptomatic bacteriuria: Host-pathogen interaction in urinary tract infections. Pediatric Nephrology 2012; DOI 10.1007/s00467-011-2089-1 http://www.springerlink.com/content/e311x5gx674hv8h8/fulltext.html

[105] Svensson M, Yadav M, Holmqvist B, Lutay N, Svanborg C, Godaly G. Acute pyelonephritis and renal scarring are caused by dysfunctional innate immunity in mCxcr2 heterozygous mice. Kidney International 2011;80(10): 1064-72. http://www.nature.com/ki/journal/v80/n10/full/ki2011257a.html

[106] Williams G, Craig JC. Prevention of recurrent urinary tract infection in children. Current Opinion in Infectious Diseases 2009;22(1): 72-6. http://journals.lww.com/co-infectiousdiseases/Abstract/2009/02000/Prevention_of_recurrent_urinary_tract_infection_in.12.aspx

Chapter 8

Immune-Based Treatment Strategies for Patients with Recurrent Urinary Tract Infections – Where Are We?

Thomas Nelius, Christopher Winter,
Julia Willingham and Stephanie Filleur

Additional information is available at the end of the chapter

http://dx.doi.org/10.5772/52913

1. Introduction

Urinary tract infections (UTI) are among the most common bacterial infections in humans. Approximately 50%-60% of adult women experience a UTI during their lifetime. Furthermore, a significant number of patients can be characterized as having recurrent UTIs if they meet the criteria of ≥2 uncomplicated UTIs in 6 months or ≥3 positive cultures within the preceding 12 months. Applying this definition, it is estimated that recurrent UTIs affect 25% of women with a history of UTI.

E. coli represents the main causative pathogen in recurrent UTI and is responsible for approximately 80% of all episodes of infection. Further important pathogens include Proteus mirabilis, Staphylococcus saprophyticus, and Klebsiella pneumonia.

Symptomatic UTIs cause significant discomfort such as dysuria, polyuria, and suprapubic tenderness. If left untreated, a UTI can progress to acute pyelonephritis with the risk of permanent renal scarring and loss of renal function.

Patients with recurrent urinary tract infections undergo frequent antibiotic treatment and/or low-dose antibiotic prophylaxis. Additionally, a subset of patients is required to undergo a systematic radiological and endoscopic evaluation of the urinary tract in order to rule out any underlying structural abnormalities or urinary calculi. The immense use of antibiotics for the treatment of urinary tract infections has resulted in the development of considerable bacterial resistance and therefore, increasing difficulties in eradicating infections. Due to the development of bacterial resistance, UTIs are a substantial economic burden and a noteworthy public health issue. Therefore, new treatment strategies and preventive measures against UTIs such as immune-stimulation/modulation, vaccine development, the use of probiotics, and the instillation of attenuated bacteria into the urinary bladder are currently being researched.

This chapter will review the most recent literature and provide up-to-date information on developments in immune-based treatment strategies for patients with recurrent UTIs from a pre-clinical and clinical point of view.

2. Material and methods

To identify all relevant materials, comprehensive literature searches were performed via the data sources: MEDLINE, EMBASE, CINAHL and OVID using the key words: urinary tract infection, urine culture, UTI, vaccines, adherence, fimbriae, biofilms, probiotics. Relevant articles and references between 1970 and 2012 were reviewed and analyzed. Reference lists from relevant review articles were also searched. Only articles published as formal papers in peer-reviewed journals were selected for inclusion if they reported findings of interest. The data base searches resulted in 710 articles, of which 75 of 710 pertained directly to immune-based treatment strategies. The entirety of these articles was reviewed, forming the basis for the current review.

3. Results

Plant-derived therapies have long been used in Ayurvedic and traditional Chinese medicine (Wollenweber, 1988). The interest in plant antimicrobials for treatment or prevention of UTIs has been driven both by the prevalence of antibiotic-resistant uropathogens and growing popularity of complementary and alternative medicine. Still, little evidence exists for the effectiveness of these treatments and therapeutic dose requirements. More than 5000 plant polyphenols have been identified so far. The spectrum of biological effects include anti-microbiol, anti-inflammatory and anti-carcinogenic activities (Beretz et al., 1978). Plant derived extracts contain different chemical compounds with multiple antimicrobial activities (Burt, 2004). The most studied species include cranberry, berberine, blueberry, bearberry, and certain herbs such as cinnamon. According to Ohno et al., the potential for bacteria to develop resistance to plant derived anti-microbials is relatively small (Ohno et al., 2003).

3.1. Cranberry

Cranberry, Vaccinium macrocapron, is the best known and most studied plant-derived therapy for UTIs (Seeram, 2008). Historically its antimicrobial effects were believed to be due increased excretion of hippuric acid and urinary acidification, although this was disproved in the 1950's (Bodel et al., 1959). More recent studies have proved Cranberry compounds fructose and proanthocyanidin to inhibit E. Coli adhesins *in vitro*. This finding has given rise to the currently held hypothesis that cranberry extracts prevent E. Coli adhesion to bladder mucosa, thus decreasing the incidence of UTIs (Howell et al., 2005, Lavigne et al., 2008, Liu et al., 2006, Ofek et al., 1991, Ohnishi et al., 2006). More recently, other compounds such as flavanoids, anthocyanins, catechin, triterpenoids, organic acids and ascorbic acid were identified as constituents (Raz et al., 2004). A wide variety of cranberry products are employed as treatment, the most common are cranberry juice concentrate, cranberry juice cocktail, and capsules. In respect to prevention, randomised trials suggest that cranberry juice or cranberry-concentrate tablets reduce the risk of symptomatic recurrent infection by 12-20%, especially in pre-menopausal women (Avorn et al., 1994, Kontiokari et al., 2001, Stothers, 2002). The same results do not apply to men, elderly patients, or those requiring catheterization (Jepson &Craig, 2008). When compared to the current standard of antibiotic treatment, trimethoprim-sulfamethoxazole 480mg daily is more effective than cranberry capsules 500mg twice daily to prevent recurrent UTIs over 12 months (Beerepoot et al.). High withdrawal rates were common in these trials, as was the inability to confirm compliance with cranberry prophylaxis. While some randomized clinical trials could not demonstrate that cranberry is beneficial (Jepson et al., 2000), other clinical and epidemiological studies support the use of cranberry in maintaining a healthy urinary tract (Perez-Lopez et al., 2009). Another proposed mode of action is the non-enzymatic generation of nitric oxide under acidic conditions(MacMicking et al., 1997). Nitric oxide has significant anti-microbial activity. Up until now, no evidence exists that cranberry extracts are effective to treat UTIs, while some data support its use as prophylactic agent in the prevention of UTIs (Guay, 2009).

3.1.1. Berberine

Berberine sulfate is an alkaloid found in the Berberine arisata plant, as well as the roots of Oregon Grape (Mahonia aquifolium), Goldenseal (hydrastis canadensis), and Goldenthread (Coptis chinesis). It is present in the root, rhizome, and stem bark of the plants (Yarnell, 2002). Head et al. could show that berberine extracts are effective against a variety of organisms, including bacteria, viruses, fungi, and protozoans (Head, 2008). Growth inhibitory effects were described for several bacterial pathogens such as Staphylococcus aureus, Pseudomonas aeruginosa,, E. coli, Bacillus subtilis and Chlamydia (Cernakova &Kostalova, 2002, Head, 2008, Scazzocchio et al., 2001). In one study berberine was found to decrease synthesis and expression of E. Coli Pap fimbriae, thus decreasing bacterial adhesion to epithelia *in vitro* (Sun et al., 1988). Similarly, berberine sulfate was found to prevent Streptococcus pyogenes to adhere to host cells (Sun et al., 1988). Another potentially important mode of action, is the alteration of the bacterial cell division through targeting the FtsZ protein (Domadia et al., 2008). However, the mechanisms behind the anti-microbial properties of berbine are not well studied. Although berberine has been included in Chinese urinary medications for centuries, no *in vivo* studies or clinical trials have been published to evaluate its effectiveness.

3.1.2. Blueberry

Blueberry, part of the Vaccinium genus, is closely related to cranberry. Studies suggest that high molecular weight pranthocyanidins found in wild blueberry inhibit E. Coli adhesion *in vitro* (Head, 2008, Ofek et al., 1996, Ofek et al., 1991). It was also shown, that the constituents in blueberry extracts similarly to those in cranberry extracts inhibit uropathogenic E. coli (UPEC) from adhering to the uroepithelial cells using the mannose-resistant adhesin. This was measured by the ability of prepared blueberry fractions to suppress the agglutination of human red blood cells after incubation with UPEC strains (Schmidt et al., 2004). No relevant trials of blueberry alone for UTI prevention or treatment were found at this time.

3.1.3. Bearberry

Bearberry, Arcystaphylos uva-ursi, is a member of the Ericaceae family, as are cranberry and blueberry. The glycoside arbutin is the main constituent of bearberry leaves and dried preparation. Arbutin is metabolized into hydroquinone, which has a urinary availability of approximately 65% of the administered arbutin dose (Schindler et al., 2002). Hydroquinone is an antimicrobial according to *in vitro* studies, although there are no *in vivo* studies to prove its effectiveness (Frohne, 1970). Turi et al. showed that growth of clinical isolates of UPEC in the presence of Arcystaphylos uva-ursi extracts change microbial cell surface characteristics by increasing the microbial cell surface hydrophobicity, thereby decreasing their ability to adhere to host cells (Turi et al., 1997). Furthermore, Arcystaphylos uva-ursi was described as diuretic and anti-inflammatory agent, effects that are supportive in the treatment of UTIs (Beaux et al., 1999, Kubo et al., 1990).

Currently, bearberry is used in Germany to cure mild UTI, defined as asymptomatic or bacteriuria less than 10^5 colony-forming units/mL (Schindler et al., 2002). It is not, however, recommended for long-term prevention due to concern of hydroquinone carcinogenic effects (DeCaprio, 1999).

3.1.4. Trans-cinnamaldehyde

Trans-cinnamaldehyde is an extract of the bark of cinnamon (Adams et al., 2004). It has a wide margin of safety between conservative estimates of intake and no observed adverse effects (Adams et al., 2004). *In vitro* studies demonstrated antibacterial activity against Clostridium botulinum, S. aureus, E. coli O157:H7 and Salmonella Typhimurium. Recently, it was shown that trans-cinnamaldehyde has the ability to inhibit UPEC biofilm formation on urinary catheters and to inhibited the adhesion and invasion of uroepithelial cells by UPEC by down regulation of major virulence genes (Amalaradjou et al.). Other antimicrobial mechanisms include changes in the permeability of cell membranes, inhibitory effects on enzymes such as amino acid decarboxylases and inhibiting the production of virulence factors (Gill &Holley, 2006, Sikkema et al., 1994, Smith-Palmer et al., 2002).

These results justify further pre-clinical studies and make trans-cinnamaldehyde a potential candidate for use as an antimicrobial agent for controlling UTIs.

3.1.5. Others

The existing literature lists many other herbs for the treatment of UTIs, while most of them lack a scientific basis for this purpose. They include Taraxacum officinalis leaf (dandelion), Juniperus communis (juniper), Hydrangea aborescens (hydrangea), Agrimonia eupatoria (agrimony), Elymus repens (couchgrass), Althea officinalis (marshmallow), Zea mays (corn silk), Apium graveolens (celery seed), Ulmus fulva (slippery elm), Arctium lappa (burdock), and Mentha piperita (peppermint). For others some scientific background exists. Extracts from Salvia officinalis (Garden sage or common sage) has been shown to be active against Klebsiella, Enterobacter species, UPEC, Proteus mirabilis and Morganella morganii obtained from the urine samples from patients with UTIs (Pereira et al., 2004).

Another potentially useful herb is Barosma betulina (bachu). It has been used in the treatment of UTI and urethritis for a long time. It was found to have anti-microbial effects against uropathogens *in vitro* and diuretic properties (Simpson, 1998).

3.2. Vaginal probiotics/lactobacilli

Studies could demonstrate that Lactobacilllus species in the form of probiotics reduced the risk of UTIs and vaginal infections (Bruce &Reid, 2003, Reid et al.,1985). However, despite ongoing research the mechanisms are poorly understood (Spiegel et al., 1980). In the literature were different mode of action proposed including downregulation of pro-inflammatory cytokines (IL-6, IL-8, TNF-alpha) (Anukam et al., 2009), production of hydrogen peroxide, which protects against the UPEC (Czaja et al., 2007) production of a 29-kDa biosurfactant proteins which inhibits bacterial adhesion (Osset et al., 2001, Xia et al., 2006). Some of the commensal bacteria such as Lactobacillus species and Bifidobacteria species are known to produce immunoregulatory factors that modulate the immune response and may therefore decrease UTIs (Wilson et al., 1998). From a clinical standpoint, there is a close correlation between loss of the normal genital microbiota, particularly Lactobacillus species, and an increased incidence of genital and bladder infections. Vaginal colonization with Lactobacillus spp. was found to prevent recurrent UTIs (Bruce &Reid, 1988, Reid et al., 1992). A Phase I clinical trial assessed the safety of the use of vaginal Lactobacillus suppositories to prevent recurrent (Czaja et al., 2007). Reid et al. investigated in a randomized study the role of probiotic lactobacilli in controlling re-infection in women after treatment of an acute UTI (Reid et al., 1992). 235 patients were treated with antibiotics for three days. Recurrence occurred in 41% of the patients. Individuals with recurrence were randomly assigned to Lactobacillus suppositories treatment group or placebo suppository group. Treatment was given twice weekly for two weeks, then once a month for the next two months. The recurrence rate was 21% in the Lactobacillus group compared to 47% in the placebo group. Oral use of Lactobacilli was also investigated. Reid et al. demonstrated L. rhamonosus GR-1 and L. fermentum RC-14 taken orally lead to colonization of vaginal epithelium within one week. In pediatric patients the oral intake of L. rhamnosus GG resulted in a reduction in UTI incidence rate compared to the placebo group (Dani et al., 2002). These results are promising and warrant further pre-clinical and clinical studies for the use of probiotics in controlling UTIs.

3.3. Immuno-stimulation/vaccines

Currently, low-dose antibiotic treatment has been the most effective prophylaxis for the prevention of recurrent UTI. However, cessation of antibiotic treatment usually results in recurrence of infection in most patients (Ha &Cho, 2008). Furthermore, with the number of antibiotic resistant strains of uropathogenic bacteria causing recurrent UTI on the rise, a substantial amount of research in alternative treatment modalities such as immuno-stimulation and attenuated vaccines is being performed. The target of such modalities consists of the Mucosa-Associated Lymphoid Tissue (MALT) lining much of the GI, respiratory, and genitourinary tract, the activation of specific receptors on dendritic cells within the genitourinary tract, and increasing the concentration bacteria-specific immunoglobulins (Ha &Cho, 2008). The objective of such therapies is to reduce the frequency and severity of UTI as well as reduce the consumption of antibiotics used to treat them.

Uro-Vaxom® (OM-89) is an extract of 18 strains of E. coli that is obtained by alkaline lysis, which destroys lipopolysaccharide (LPS) molecules produced by the gram negative bacteria and modifies other bacterial antigens, maintaining their antigenic potential (Ha &Cho, 2008). Taken orally, Uro-Vaxom® achieves immuno-stimulation by increasing the proliferation of Mucosal Associated Lymphoid Tissue (MALT) within the GI tract leading to elevated concentrations of bacteria-specific IgG, mucosal-derived IgA along with serum IgA. Furthermore, OM-89 increases the rate of dendritic cell maturation within the genitourinary tract, leading to increased numbers of circulating memory T-cells as well as an overall increase in inflammatory mediators such as TNF-alpha, IL-2, and IL-6 (Bessler et al., 2009). Treatment studies of sexually active females between the age of 20 and 50 shows that Uro-Vaxom® reduces the recurrence of UTI by 36% after 6 months of therapy compared to placebo (Bessler et al., 2009).

Solco Urovac, which is currently under phase 2 clinical trials, is a treatment modality that utilizes the vaginal mucosa via suppository to induce an immune response. The Solco Urovac vaccine consists of 6 E. coli strains along with several recombinant antigenic factors such as fimbriae proteins and 1 strain each of Proteus mirabilis, Morganella morganii, Klebsiella pneumonia, and Enterococcus faecalis (Hopkins et al., 2007). SolcoUrovac works in a similar manner to that of OM-89, however it achieves a higher overall mucosal concentration of IgA in the vagina and bladder. One characteristic of SolcoUrovac is that it must be administered on a booster schedule or else the maximum efficacy will not be achieved. The overall reduction of UTIs in female patients between the age of late teens to early 70s treated with SolcoUrovac plus multiple boosters was measured to be 46.0% (Hopkins et al., 2007).

Siderophores, such as the IroN-cell surface protein found on most strains of E. Coli, are potential targets for immune-therapy. A significant systemic-compartment IroN IgG-specific antibody response developed in serum. However, there was no IroN IgA-specific antibody response in either the systemic or the mucosal compartment. Subcutaneous immunization with denatured IroN resulted in a significant IroN immunoglobulin G (IgG)-specific response in serum but not a systemic or mucosal IroN-specific IgA response (Russo et al., 2003).

3.4. Inhibition of bacterial adhesion

UPEC strains express a number of virulence factors used for colonization of their host. One important virulence factor is located on type 1 pili, allowing UPEC to adhere and invade host cells within the urinary tract. FimH interactions with several host factors have been documented. These include components of the glycocalyx that sparsely covers the bladder surface, carcinoembryonic antigen-related cell adhesion molecule (CEACAM) family members, soluble Tamm-Horsfall protein, the glycosylphosphatidylinositol (GPI)-anchored protein CD48, the leukocyte adhesion molecules CD11 and CD18, and uroplakin 1a (Klein et al.). Adherence to mannose residues prevents the rapid clearance of E. coli from the urinary tract by the flow of urine and enables the invasion of the host cells (Wellens et al., 2008). The binding of type one pili to bladder epithelial cells activates the innate immune system via the Toll-like receptor 4 pathway which recruits neutrophils and other inflammatory mediators to the site of insult (Wellens et al., 2008). Next, the complement system opsonizes the UPEC and counter intuitively facilitates invasion of the bacteria into the epithelial cell.

Type 1 pili are the most prevalent fimbriae encoded by UPEC, consisting of the four subunits FimA, FimF, FimG, and FimH, the latter located at the tip of the pili (Wellens et al., 2008). The FimH moiety, which is the primarily subunit responsible for the initiation of bacterial adherence and invasion, is a prime target of immune-stimulation. Experiments done in mice have shown that both direct inoculation with immunogloblins against FimH, innoculation with synthetic peptides within the binding moiety for FimH, or gene knock-out of FimH could specifically block type 1 fimbriae-mediated bacterial adherence to bladder epithelial cells resulting in a dramatic loss of virulence(Thankavel et al., 1997). In experiments that utilized synthetic peptides to induce an immune response, dramatic increases in serum IgG and IgM were observed via ELISA (Thankavel et al., 1997). In addition, urine collections showed a marked increase in IgG and mucosal derived IgA along with elevated activity of mast cells within the bladder epithelium when faced with a bacterial challenge (Thankavel et al., 1997).

3.5. Inhibition of bacterial biofilms

Catheter–associated urinary tract infections are common and often related to the existence of bacterial bio-films. Progress in this area is limited. Preventive strategies include avoiding unnecessary catheterization, limit duration of catheterization, using closed drainage system, and appropriate hygiene, including frequent catheter changes and emptying of the drainage bags (Jacobsen et al., 2008, Newman, 1998). Many mechanisms of biofilm resistance against antibiotic treatment were reported over the years. The most important type of the biofilm resistance is the development of a diffusion barrier formed by the bio-film matrix (Ishida et al., 1998). The biofilm prevents access of antimicrobial agents and even of antibodies. Despite the antibiotic treatment, the infection often persists until the device is removed (Schierholz &Beuth, 2001). Over the last 2 decades different coatings were explored to reduce the risk of bacterial bio-film formation and bacterial colonization and subsequently infection. Coating substances included various antibiotics, silvercoating and others. Infections could not be prevented, however the "abacterial window" could be prolonged. Schaeffer et al. demonstrated that in patients with acute spinal cord injury, who received long-term urinary catheters, the silver-coated catheters delayed but did not prevent the onset of bacteriuria (Schaeffer et al., 1988). The same findings were reported for antibiotic impregnation of catheters (Darouiche et al., 1999, Guay, 2001, Johnson et al., 1999). These findings are important for short-term use of urinary catheters but not for long-term use (Trautner &Darouiche, 2004). Several other substances were reported to inhibit development of bacterial bio-film formation including type A proanthocyanidins, hesperidin, apigenin,naringin and rhoifolina, and others. None of these substances made it into clinical trials so far.

3.6. Stimulation of cyclic adenosine/forskolin

One important survival mechanism of UPEC is the creation of an intracellular reservoir. Within the epithelial cell, the UPEC are able to resist antibiotic treatment by binding to Rab 27 b/CD 63 positive vesicles. Forskolin, the active component of the Coleus forskohlii, has been proven to increase the content of cyclical adenosine monophosphate (cAMP) in urothelial cells, leading uropathogenic bacteria to exit the urothelial cells. It was shown that cAMP levels regulate the exocytosis of these vesicles depending on the bladder distension. These findings could lead to new approaches for the treatment and prevention of recurrent urinary tract infections (Bishop et al., 2007, Gonzalez-Chamorro et al.).

3.7. Hormone therapy

Hormonal deficiency in postmenopausal women results in thinning of the vaginal and urethral mucosa and more importantly to disruption of the normal vaginal flora and therefore to an increased risk for UTIs (Head, 2008). Several studies could demonstrate, that replacing estrogene in this patient population can reduce the incidence of UTIs.

In a randomized study postmenopausal women received either intra-vaginally administered estradiol or placebo. At the end of the study a significant reduction in the incidence of UTIs in the treatment group compared to the placebo group was noted. Of interest is also the observation that Lactobacilli that were absent in the vaginal cultures of patients of the treatment group at the beginning of the trial reappeared in 61% (Raz &Stamm, 1993).

3.8. Instillation of attenuated bacteria into the urinary bladder

Darouiche et al. conducted a prospective, randomized, placebo-controlled, double-blind pilot trial to examine the efficacy of bacterial interference in preventing urinary tract infection (Darouiche et al., 2005). In this study 27 patients with spinal cord injury were included. Patients were randomly assigned either to have their bladders inoculated with either E. coli 83972 (experimental group) or sterile normal saline (control group). Patients whose bladders became colonized with E. coli 83972 were half as likely (P=.01) than non-colonized patients to develop UTI during the subsequent year.

Billips et al. demonstrated recently that deletion of the O antigen ligase gene, waaL, from the uropathogenic E. coli isolate NU14 results in a strain that stimulates enhanced urothelial cytokine secretion (Billips et al., 2009). They could show that NU14 DwaaL stimulated an enhanced interleukin-6 secretion by mouse macrophages, compared with secretion by the wild type. Of great importance is the fact that mice vaccinated via instillation into the bladder developed protective responses that prevented persistent colonization after bladder challenge with NU14, yet NU14 DwaaL failed to persistently colonize the mouse bladder. They could

http://dx.doi.org/10.5772/52913

also show that the mice were additionally protected against challenge with a broad range of clinical UPEC isolates and developed immunity that lasted more than 8 weeks (Billips et al., 2009). These findings open a new avenue for future treatment strategies of recurrent urinary tract infection by caused by UPEC.

4. Discussion

Immune-based treatment strategies for patients with recurrent UTIs are of special interest. Several promising new approaches including bladder colonization with attenuated bacteria and intravesical vaccination were published recently and discussed in this chapter. Furthermore, studies suggest that the use of inhibitors of bacterial adherence to urothelial cell and inhibitors of biofilm formation receptors hold great promise. Moreover, stimulators of cyclic AMP inside urothelial cells and the recent advancements in the development of vaccines are an interesting initiative in this field. For some of the plant –based prevention and treatment strategies only little scientific evidence for the prevention and treatment of urinary tract infection exist.

Acknowledgment

We would like to thank the library staff from Texas Tech University Health Sciences Center, Lubbock for their extraordinary support and assistance. On a special note, we would like to thank again Carrie Gassett who showed great interest and support in our project.

Author details

Thomas Nelius, Christopher Winter, Julia Willingham and Stephanie Filleur

Texas Tech University Health Sciences Center, Departments of Urology and Microbiology, Lubbock, USA

References

[1] Adams, T. B., et al. (2004). The FEMA GRAS assessment of cinnamyl derivatives used as flavor ingredients. Food Chem Toxicol, Feb 2004), Print), 42(2), 157-185.

[2] Amalaradjou, M. A., Narayanan, A. ., & Venkitanarayanan, K. Trans-cinnamaldehyde decreases attachment and invasion of uropathogenic Escherichia coli in urinary

tract epithelial cells by modulating virulence gene expression. J Urol, Apr Electronic), 185(4), 1526-1531.

[3] Anukam, K. C., et al. (2009). Probiotic Lactobacillus rhamnosus GR-1 and Lactobacillus reuteri RC-14 may help downregulate TNF-Alpha, IL-6, IL-8, IL-10 and IL-12 (p70) in the neurogenic bladder of spinal cord injured patient with urinary tract infections: a two-case study. Adv Urol, Vol. Print)(2009), 680363.

[4] Avorn, J., et al. (1994). Reduction of bacteriuria and pyuria after ingestion of cranberry juice. Jama, Mar 9 1994), Print), 271(10), 751-754.

[5] Beaux, D., Fleurentin, J. ., & Mortier, F. (1999). Effect of extracts of Orthosiphon stamineus Benth, Hieracium pilosella L., Sambucus nigra L. and Arctostaphylos uva-ursi (L.) Spreng. in rats. Phytother Res, May 1999), X (Print), 13(3), 222-225.

[6] Beerepoot, M. A., et al. Cranberries vs antibiotics to prevent urinary tract infections: a randomized double-blind noninferiority trial in premenopausal women. Arch Intern Med, Jul 25 Electronic), 171(14), 1270-1278.

[7] Beretz, A., Anton, R. ., & Stoclet, J. C. (1978). Flavonoid compounds are potent inhibitors of cyclic AMP phosphodiesterase. ExperientiaAug 15 1978), Print), 34(8), 1054-1055.

[8] Bessler, W. G., et al. (2009). Immunomodulating effects of OM-89, a bacterial extract from Escherichia coli, in murine and human leukocytes. Arzneimittelforschung, Print), 59(11), 571-577.

[9] Billips, B. K., et al. (2009). A live-attenuated vaccine for the treatment of urinary tract infection by uropathogenic Escherichia coli. J Infect Dis, Jul 15 2009), Print), 200(2), 263-272.

[10] Bishop, B. L., et al. (2007). Cyclic AMP-regulated exocytosis of Escherichia coli from infected bladder epithelial cells. Nat Med, May 2007), Print), 13(5), 625-630.

[11] Bodel, P. T., Cotran, R. ., & Kass, E. H. (1959). Cranberry juice and the antibacterial action of hippuric acid. J Lab Clin Med, No. (Dec 1959), Print), 54, 881-888.

[12] Bruce, A. W. ., & Reid, G. (1988). Intravaginal instillation of lactobacilli for prevention of recurrent urinary tract infections. Can J Microbiol, Mar 1988), , 34(3), 339-343.

[13] Bruce, A. W. ., & Reid, G. (2003). Probiotics and the urologist. Can J Urol, Apr 2003), , 10(2), 1785-1789.

[14] Burt, S. (2004). Essential oils: their antibacterial properties and potential applications in foods--a review. Int J Food Microbiol, Aug 1 2004), Print), 94(3), 223-253.

[15] Cernakova, M. ., & Kostalova, D. (2002). Antimicrobial activity of berberine--a constituent of Mahonia aquifolium. Folia Microbiol (Praha), Print), 47(4), 375-378.

[16] Czaja, C. A., et al. (2007). Phase I trial of a Lactobacillus crispatus vaginal suppository for prevention of recurrent urinary tract infection in women. Infect Dis Obstet Gynecol, , 2007(2007), 35387.

[17] Dani, C., et al. (2002). Probiotics feeding in prevention of urinary tract infection, bacterial sepsis and necrotizing enterocolitis in preterm infants. A prospective double-blind study. Biol Neonate, Aug 2002), , 82(2), 103-108.

[18] Darouiche, R. O., et al. (1999). Efficacy of antimicrobial-impregnated bladder catheters in reducing catheter-associated bacteriuria: a prospective, randomized, multicenter clinical trial. UrologyDec 1999), Electronic), 54(6), 976-981.

[19] Darouiche, R. O., et al. (2005). Bacterial interference for prevention of urinary tract infection: a prospective, randomized, placebo-controlled, double-blind pilot trial. Clin Infect Dis, Nov 15 2005), Electronic), 41(10), 1531-1534.

[20] De Caprio, A. P. (1999). The toxicology of hydroquinone--relevance to occupational and environmental exposure. Crit Rev Toxicol, May 1999), Print), 29(3), 283-330.

[21] Domadia, P. N., et al. (2008). Berberine targets assembly of Escherichia coli cell division protein FtsZ. BiochemistryMar 11 2008), Print), 47(10), 3225-3234.

[22] Frohne, D. (1970). The urinary disinfectant effect of extract from leaves uva ursi]. Planta Med, Jan 1970), Print), 18(1), 1-25.

[23] Gill, A O &Holley, R A.(2006). Disruption of Escherichia coli, Listeria monocytogenes and Lactobacillus sakei cellular membranes by plant oil aromatics. Int J Food Microbiol, Apr 15 2006), Print), 108(1), 1-9.

[24] Gonzalez-Chamorro, F., & et, al. [. Urinary tract infections and their prevention]. Actas Urol Esp, Jan Electronic), 36(1), 48-53.

[25] Guay, D. R. (2009). Cranberry and urinary tract infections. Drugs, Print), 69(7), 775-807.

[26] Guay, D. R. (2001). An update on the role of nitrofurans in the management of urinary tract infections. Drugs, Print), 61(3), 353-364.

[27] Ha, U S &Cho, Y H.(2008). Immunostimulation with Escherichia coli extract: prevention of recurrent urinary tract infections. Int J Antimicrob Agents, Suppl 1, No. (Feb 2008), Print), 31, S63-S67.

[28] Head, K. A. (2008). Natural approaches to prevention and treatment of infections of the lower urinary tract. Altern Med Rev, Sep 2008), Print), 13(3), 227-244.

[29] Hopkins, W. J., et al. (2007). Vaginal mucosal vaccine for recurrent urinary tract infections in women: results of a phase 2 clinical trial. J Urol, Apr 2007), quiz 1591, 0022-5347 (Print), 177(4), 1349-1353.

[30] Howell, A. B., et al. (2005). A-type cranberry proanthocyanidins and uropathogenic bacterial anti-adhesion activity. Phytochemistry, Sep 2005), Print), 66(18), 2281-2291.

[31] Ishida, H., et al. (1998). In vitro and in vivo activities of levofloxacin against biofilm-producing Pseudomonas aeruginosa. Antimicrob Agents Chemother, Jul 1998), Print), 42(7), 1641-1645.

[32] Jacobsen, S. M., et al. (2008). Complicated catheter-associated urinary tract infections due to Escherichia coli and Proteus mirabilis. Clin Microbiol Rev, Jan 2008), Electronic), 21(1), 26-59.

[33] Jepson, R G &Craig, J C.(2008). Cranberries for preventing urinary tract infections. Cochrane Database Syst Rev, Vol. X (Electronic)(1), CD001321.

[34] Jepson, R. G., Mihaljevic, L. ., & Craig, J. (2000). Cranberries for treating urinary tract infections. Cochrane Database Syst Rev, Vol. X (Electronic)(2), CD001322.

[35] Johnson, J. R., Delavari, P. ., & Azar, M. (1999). Activities of a nitrofurazone-containing urinary catheter and a silver hydrogel catheter against multidrug-resistant bacteria characteristic of catheter-associated urinary tract infection. Antimicrob Agents Chemother, Dec 1999), Print), 43(12), 2990-2995.

[36] Klein, T et al. FimH antagonists for the oral treatment of urinary tract infections: from design and synthesis to in vitro and in vivo evaluation. J Med Chem, Vol. 53, No. 24, (Dec 23 pp. 8627-8641, 1520-4804 (Electronic)

[37] Kontiokari, T., et al. (2001). Randomised trial of cranberry-lingonberry juice and Lactobacillus GG drink for the prevention of urinary tract infections in women. Bmj, Jun 30 2001), Print), 322(7302), 1571.

[38] Kubo, M., et al. (1990). Pharmacological studies on leaf of Arctostaphylos uva-ursi (L.) Spreng. I. Combined effect of 50% methanolic extract from Arctostaphylos uva-ursi (L.) Spreng. (bearberry leaf) and prednisolone on immuno-inflammation]. Yakugaku Zasshi, Jan 1990), Print), 110(1), 59-67.

[39] Lavigne, J. P., et al. (2008). In-vitro and in-vivo evidence of dose-dependent decrease of uropathogenic Escherichia coli virulence after consumption of commercial Vaccinium macrocarpon (cranberry) capsules. Clin Microbiol Infect, Apr 2008), X (Print), 14(4), 350-355.

[40] Liu, Y., et al. (2006). Role of cranberry juice on molecular-scale surface characteristics and adhesion behavior of Escherichia coli. Biotechnol Bioeng, Feb 5 2006), Print), 93(2), 297-305.

[41] Mac, Micking. J., Xie, Q. W. ., & Nathan, C. (1997). Nitric oxide and macrophage function. Annu Rev Immunol, Print), 15(1997), 323-350.

[42] Newman, D. K. (1998). Managing indwelling urethral catheters. Ostomy Wound Manage, Dec 1998), passim, 0889-5899 (Print), 44(12), 26-28.

[43] Ofek, I., Goldhar, J. ., & Sharon, N. (1996). Anti-Escherichia coli adhesin activity of cranberry and blueberry juices. Adv Exp Med Biol, Print), 408(1996), 179-183.

[44] Ofek, I., et al. (1991). Anti-Escherichia coli adhesin activity of cranberry and blueberry juices. N Engl J Med, May 30 1991), Print), 324(22), 1599.

[45] Ohnishi, R., et al. (2006). Urinary excretion of anthocyanins in humans after cranberry juice ingestion. Biosci Biotechnol Biochem, Jul 2006), Print), 70(7), 1681-1687.

[46] Ohno, T., et al. (2003). Antimicrobial activity of essential oils against Helicobacter pylori. Helicobacter, Jun 2003), Print), 8(3), 207-215.

[47] Osset, J., et al. (2001). Assessment of the capacity of Lactobacillus to inhibit the growth of uropathogens and block their adhesion to vaginal epithelial cells. J Infect Dis, Feb 1 2001), , 183(3), 485-491.

[48] Pereira, R. S., et al. (2004). Antibacterial activity of essential oils on microorganisms isolated from urinary tract infection]. Rev Saude Publica, Apr 2004), , 38(2), 326-328.

[49] Perez-Lopez, F. R., Haya, J. ., & Chedraui, P. (2009). Vaccinium macrocarpon: an interesting option for women with recurrent urinary tract infections and other health benefits. J Obstet Gynaecol Res, Aug 2009), Print), 35(4), 630-639.

[50] Raz, R., Chazan, B. ., & Dan, M. (2004). Cranberry juice and urinary tract infection. Clin Infect Dis, May 15 2004), Electronic), 38(10), 1413-1419.

[51] Raz, R. ., & Stamm, W. E. (1993). A controlled trial of intravaginal estriol in postmenopausal women with recurrent urinary tract infections. N Engl J Med, Sep 9 1993), Print), 329(11), 753-756.

[52] Reid, G., Bruce, A. W. ., & Taylor, M. (1992). Influence of three-day antimicrobial therapy and lactobacillus vaginal suppositories on recurrence of urinary tract infections. Clin Ther, Jan-Feb 1992), , 14(1), 11-16.

[53] Reid, G., et al. (1985). Prevention of urinary tract infection in rats with an indigenous Lactobacillus casei strain. Infect Immun, Aug 1985), , 49(2), 320-324.

[54] Russo, T. A., et al. (2003). The Siderophore receptor IroN of extraintestinal pathogenic Escherichia coli is a potential vaccine candidate. Infect Immun, Dec 2003), Print), 71(12), 7164-7169.

[55] Scazzocchio, F., et al. (2001). Antibacterial activity of Hydrastis canadensis extract and its major isolated alkaloids. Planta Med, Aug 2001), Print), 67(6), 561-564.

[56] Schaeffer, A. J., Story, K. O. ., & Johnson, S. M. (1988). Effect of silver oxide/trichloroisocyanuric acid antimicrobial urinary drainage system on catheter-associated bacteriuria. J Urol, Jan 1988), Print), 139(1), 69-73.

[57] Schierholz, J. M. ., & Beuth, J. (2001). Implant infections: a haven for opportunistic bacteria. J Hosp Infect, Oct 2001), Print), 49(2), 87-93.

[58] Schindler, G., et al. (2002). Urinary excretion and metabolism of arbutin after oral administration of Arctostaphylos uvae ursi extract as film-coated tablets and aqueous solution in healthy humans. J Clin Pharmacol, Aug 2002), Print), 42(8), 920-927.

[59] Schmidt, B. M., et al. (2004). Effective separation of potent antiproliferation and antiadhesion components from wild blueberry (Vaccinium angustifolium Ait.) fruits. J Agric Food Chem, Oct 20 2004), Print), 52(21), 6433-6442.

[60] Seeram, N. P. (2008). Berry fruits for cancer prevention: current status and future prospects. J Agric Food Chem, Feb 13 2008), Print), 56(3), 630-635.

[61] Sikkema, J;de., Bont, J. A. ., & Poolman, B. (1994). Interactions of cyclic hydrocarbons with biological membranes. J Biol Chem, Mar 18 1994), Print), 269(11), 8022-8028.

[62] Simpson, D. (1998). Buchu--South Africa's amazing herbal remedy. Scott Med J, Dec 1998), , 43(6), 189-191.

[63] Smith-Palmer, A., Stewartt, J. ., & Fyfe, L. (2002). Inhibition of listeriolysin O and phosphatidylcholine-specific production in Listeria monocytogenes by subinhibitory concentrations of plant essential oils. J Med Microbiol, Jul 2002), , 51(7), 567-574.

[64] Spiegel, C. A., et al. (1980). Anaerobic bacteria in nonspecific vaginitis. N Engl J Med, Sep 11 1980), , 303(11), 601-607.

[65] Stothers, L. (2002). A randomized trial to evaluate effectiveness and cost effectiveness of naturopathic cranberry products as prophylaxis against urinary tract infection in women. Can J Urol, Jun 2002), Print), 9(3), 1558-1562.

[66] Sun, D., Abraham, S. N. ., & Beachey, E. H. (1988). Influence of berberine sulfate on synthesis and expression of Pap fimbrial adhesin in uropathogenic Escherichia coli. Antimicrob Agents Chemother, Aug 1988), Print), 32(8), 1274-1277.

[67] Sun, D., Courtney, H. S. ., & Beachey, E. H. (1988). Berberine sulfate blocks adherence of Streptococcus pyogenes to epithelial cells, fibronectin, and hexadecane. Antimicrob Agents Chemother, Sep 1988), Print), 32(9), 1370-1374.

[68] Thankavel, K., et al. (1997). Localization of a domain in the FimH adhesin of Escherichia coli type 1 fimbriae capable of receptor recognition and use of a domain-specific antibody to confer protection against experimental urinary tract infection. J Clin Invest, Sep 1 1997), Print), 100(5), 1123-1136.

[69] Trautner, B W &Darouiche, R O.(2004). Catheter-associated infections: pathogenesis affects prevention. Arch Intern Med, Apr 26 2004), Print), 164(8), 842-850.

[70] Turi, M., et al. (1997). Influence of aqueous extracts of medicinal plants on surface hydrophobicity of Escherichia coli strains of different origin. Apmis, Dec 1997), Print), 105(12), 956-962.

[71] Wellens, A., et al. (2008). Intervening with urinary tract infections using anti-adhesives based on the crystal structure of the FimH-oligomannose-3 complex. PLoS One, Electronic), 3(4), e2040.

[72] Wilson, M., Seymour, R. ., & Henderson, B. (1998). Bacterial perturbation of cytokine networks. Infect Immun, Jun 1998), , 66(6), 2401-2409.

[73] Wollenweber, E. (1988). Occurrence of flavonoid aglycones in medicinal plants. Prog Clin Biol Res, Print), 280(1988), 45-55.

[74] Xia, Y., Yamagata, K. ., & Krukoff, T. L. (2006). Differential expression of the CD14/TLR4 complex and inflammatory signaling molecules following i.c.v. administration of LPS. Brain Res, Jun 20 2006), , 1095(1), 85-95.

[75] Yarnell, E. (2002). Botanical medicines for the urinary tract. World J Urol, Nov 2002), Print), 20(5), 285-293.